MW01278576

asthma
Cured

asthma *Cured*

A Breath by Breath Journey to Health

Mavreen Jones

Copyright © 2016 by Mavreen Jones

All rights reserved. No part of this publication may be reproduced, stored in or introduced into a retrieval system, or transmitted, in any form, or by any means (electronic, mechanical, photocopying, recording or otherwise) without the prior written permission of the publisher. This book is sold subject to the condition that it shall not, by way of trade or otherwise, be lent, resold, hired out, or otherwise circulated without the publisher's prior consent in any form of binding or cover other than that in which it is published and without a similar condition including this condition being imposed on the subsequent purchaser.

Book Cover Design: Marla Thompson

Typeset: Greg Salisbury

Portrait Photographer: Natasha Jones

DISCLAIMER: The author offers this work as an additional light on asthma. This work does not constitute a healing of any type, either spiritual, emotional, or physical. Please see your medical advisor for any medical conditions you may have. Please see your spiritual advisor for any emotional, psychological, or spiritual dilemmas.

This book is dedicated to the medical profession, for without their knowledge and expertise, I would not be alive today.

It is also dedicated to the people who have discovered the ancient, natural forms of healing.

This combination of medical and natural healing has brought me to where I am today; free of asthma.

Testimonial

"aSTHMA CURED *is a welcome new voice of hope on the journey to wellness. Mavreen is living testimony to her success in conquering asthma and consequently, being healed. An insightful, stimulating and thought provoking book.*"
Wendy Edwards, Author: *It's All About Love*

"*Mavreen shows us all through her health journey, how changing your story can change your health. I have been teaching this concept for 25 years and the importance of listening to and working with your body in order to gain clarity and confidence and embody the reality that we are the authors of our own destiny. Mavreen shares how she has applied this process to heal herself and her experience serves as a reminder to all of us of what we have the power to do.*"
Dr Manon Bolliger N.D., Author: *What Patients Don't Say If Doctors Don't Ask*

"*It is my pleasure to endorse Mavreen's book* aSTHMA CURED *as a recommended book on everyone's list. I particularly enjoy her writing approach by including much of her personal story, which takes it out of the realm of theory and makes it practical. A very good book.*"
Colin P. Sisson, Author: *Rebirthing Made Easy* **and** *Inner Adventures*

Acknowledgements

It was many years ago when my friend Rita said, 'you should write a book'.

Why it has taken so long to get to this point is like wondering why no two snowflakes are the same; there is no real explanation.

Along the way I have had support about the rightness of publishing this book from many people and my staunchest supporter has been my son, Brett, who lived through that life changing era with me.

My gratitude also goes out to Wendy, an author herself, who helped me through my times of self-doubt and indecision.

Being somewhat computer challenged, I thank my friend Diane for her eleventh hour help in unscrambling something I had scrambled and could not fix.

Contents

Prologue

FROM

Allowing Sickness To Hamper My Aliveness

TO

Aliveness Sparkles Through Healing Major Ailment

Preface

After an asthma attack that almost cost me my life, I decided that I did not want to spend the rest of my life just controlling or managing the asthma by continually taking medication; my desire was to be free of asthma altogether.

My journey of discovery has brought me to that point. I have been asthma free since 1990. Because of my success in this endeavor I have written this book to share with other asthmatics and anyone who is any way involved with the illness, just how I went about doing that. The information may inspire you to begin your own personal journey to see what you can discover.

Just as the butterfly symbolizes transformation of the self, so does healing and a good place to start is with the way we think. We have the ability to know our minds and to change our minds.

Change your mind and your body will follow.

Chapter 1

THE COMA

"We are going to take you somewhere we can help you Mrs...." I hear the voice as if it's coming from out there...far away somewhere. The pain is so bad...I can't breathe...my lungs feel as if they are going to burst...my head is pounding. In response to the voice, I lift my head and open my eyes. I can't see...everything is a faint blur...it suddenly dawns on me that I am dying! I remember now...all the senses go, one by one and the hearing is the last to go...I wait for the fear to come... it doesn't matter...I have to get away from the pain...it's too much...I've never been this far before and I don't know what happens next...I've lost control! Those were my last conscious thoughts many years ago before I slipped into an unconscious state and my life changed forever.

What happened next is that I was rushed from the Emergency ward to the ICU and hooked up to life support machines. For the next four days doctors tried to stop the asthma attack I was having and they put me into an induced coma. This period was the most difficult for the doctors, my husband and fifteen year old son as I was not expected to survive.

By contrast those 4 days were the easiest for me because

I simply left my body and had the adventure of a lifetime. Whether I stayed out for the entire time I was in the coma or for just a portion of it, I don't know. Time out there doesn't relate the same to time here. A year here is like the snap of the fingers there.

There are conflicting opinions on Out of Body Experiences; about whether it does actually happen or whether the drugs cause an altered state. My feeling is that the only person who can know for sure is the one having the experience. Prior to this event, I had read many accounts of OBE's and thought I could imagine what it would be like. Not so! My imagination didn't even come close to the actual reality.

My first sensation was one of freedom which came upon me as soon as I exited the body. What came to mind at that moment was the saying....

Free at last...

Free at last...

Thank God I'm free at last!

Then there's this wonderful feeling of love. It's everywhere, all around you. Nothing on this earth compares to it. It is simply out of this world; literally. I came to realize that I was experiencing unconditional love and realized we have a long way to go in our world before we reach this state. There was no fear about being out of my body; it felt quite natural. I was aware my form was different as I wasn't tall, short, thin or fat and although I could see myself I knew I didn't have eyes as we know them. My form was like a wispy cloud that moved gently, constantly changing shape. It was similar to the Aurora Borealis that I have seen at night in the northern hemisphere. I was huge; I was an energy mass.

My thinking was the biggest surprise. I found that I had the capacity to know everything. It was quite incredible and fascinating at the same time. I remember having fun, randomly thinking about the U.S President's by number and having the name of the person come to me instantly. Today I still need to look up that information just as I did before this experience.

If I thought of a particular destination, I was instantly there. I glimpsed the future and it was clear that my dad was going to die soon, in like the time it takes to snap your fingers and I knew I had to go home to see him as soon as possible. (He was in Australia and I was living in Canada). He was healthy at that time but passed away suddenly fifteen months later and I did visit with him before that happened.

Another realization I had was that none of the things we think are important, actually are. Take for instance, our careers and our material possessions, the important meetings we must attend, the social engagements we dare not miss. None of it matters one little bit. Life is a movie, on the biggest screen of all and we are all the actors and actresses playing out our roles. What an eye opener that was for me. I realize that this concept might be hard, if not impossible, for people to grasp and I am not sure if I would have been able to, without the experience of viewing it from outside the body.

There was also a meeting with an energy mass that I recognized. When in the body this soul had been my neighbor and a surrogate grandpa to me for the first eight years of my life. When he died I was devastated and his death left a hole in my life for a long time. This time we talked telepathically and he was very loving, trying to help me realize why I was there and to decide what I was going to do next. I wasn't advised to return to my body but by looking at my life up to that point and where I was in my growth as a person, it was clear from *out there* what had to happen next and I came to my own conclusions.

I gradually became aware that there is no judgement as we know it. There is just an awareness of one's life and a knowingness of where we may have done a lot better. No one came to judge me. I was judging myself and my actions in this life and that is a lot tougher than having someone else point out your shortcomings, because when you are your own judge you have to take responsibility for the way your life has gone so far.   This reality I was in was very loving and wonderful and I had no desire to leave.

However, the longer I was there, the stronger the feeling became that I must return to my body, along with the realization that I still had things to do here on earth and that is what motivated my return.

Once I decided on my course of action, things moved very fast. I was aware of being told to hurry, to get back to the body. I suddenly found myself looking down on my body and wondering how on earth I was going to get back in because I was huge, much too big for the body.

No sooner was that thought formed than my energy mass shrank to resemble the shape of a pencil and I started moving back in, through the top of my head. About halfway in I became aware of someone moaning and I thought "Oh that poor person"…and then, click, I was back in and realized it was myself that I had heard moaning. My next impression was shock at how heavy and thick my body felt; like a lead weight* I was filled with amazement that we can actually stand our bodies upright and move them around. They are quite a dense mass. Then I opened my eyes and asked, "What happened?" At the same time I knew that I did not need to ask that question because I was quite aware of what had just happened.

*It should be noted that by this time my weight had dropped considerably, from 126lbs (57 kg) to 104 lbs. (47 kg), not exactly a lead weight

Chapter 2

LOOKING FOR ANSWERS

The events of the preceding pages created a turning point in many areas of my life and it made me all the more determined to find the root cause of the asthma. My childhood years in Australia were filled with having lots of exposure to asthma tablets, medicines and injections, all part of a search for a cure. I originally thought this was from age five onwards but my journey discovered an even earlier beginning.

At that time, England was the country where many of the medical breakthroughs were happening with asthma. Every time something new was developed I would go into the doctor's office to try the new tablets or an actual medicine that you took by the dose or perhaps receive a course of injections. Some of these caused nausea, skin irritations or in the case of the pills, really didn't help the attack but made your system speed up; much like having too much caffeine. These days medication is much different; with reliever medications (bronchodilators) for short term relief and controller medications to continually help the condition; all life-saving and very necessary for those suffering with asthma.

However, that was then and this is now; a lifetime ago in terms of how to treat asthma. Today, if you are a seeker and looking for new or different answers to the same old questions, there are ways you can do this. We are all incredible beings with a great capacity to help ourselves; we just need a nudge sometimes to get started because somewhere along the line we fell "asleep" and decided that others, not us, had all the answers. However, it doesn't have to stay that way as we are in charge of our own lives and there is a need for us to listen to what our bodies are telling us. A decision to make changes may well be the beginning of a whole new way of life towards improved health.

Some of my early findings indicated that sickness and disease can be more of a blessing than a curse and at first this did not make any sense to me at all but after my spell in the hospital I was able to see there was truth to that statement. Serious illness is like a two by four up the side of the head; it finally gets your attention, and when it gets to be as serious as what I went through, the body is literally screaming for help and asking for something to be done…or else! (and I came close to getting the "or else")

There is also a belief that we get signs along the way that the body needs help; that it is struggling, but so often we ignore them; get medication to suppress and just carry on hoping that whatever it is, will clear up. I had signs, lots of them, but ignored them all; hence the two by four. It was some time after that when I realized the blessing in all of it. It changed my life; something which was long overdue and which, for one reason or another (mainly my belief systems), I thought I was not able to do.

For each person the path to wellness will be particular to them. It may be a lot quicker, simpler and easier than mine because we each, as individuals, are different and so shall our journeys be. But whatever you do, however much time it takes you and how much success you have, it will be right for you.

Before the attack I was already trying all sorts of different techniques as I've believed, ever since I had a rare insight around the age of five or six, that, contrary to popular belief, asthma can be cured. It has not happened as yet for the masses but there may be other individuals out there, like myself, who have engineered their own cure and are just quietly getting on with life. There does seem to be some resistance in certain quarters if 'cures' are not scientifically proven which is a shame on us as a race, because learning to work together for the common cause could well be one of the reasons for us being here.

I read something years ago that has always remained with me because somehow it made perfect sense. It had to do with the idea that everything we need for our experience and survival here on earth is provided. As illness is apparently a part of our experience here, or we have made it so, then maybe the means to cure it is here too. We just have to find what that is and perhaps this is part of our personal journey.

From my own experience I found that some effort on our part is required; there is no quick fix. Modern medicine is the closest thing we have come to in that area and it does not always have the answers either. What if we started combining modern medicine with natural healing, using what works best from both and coming up with a winning combination? After all, natural healing has been around since the beginning of mankind's habitation of this planet, whereas the medical field is a relatively new one in comparison. Medically we have advanced healing in many incredible ways in a fairly short time so if the two were able to find a way to work side by side, the results may be even better than what we are getting now. The possibilities may be endless.

I wonder too, if perhaps it is time we all started looking at ways in which we help ourselves instead of waiting for someone else to fix us. Perhaps the time has come for us to take responsibility for the asthma and start to ask ourselves, 'What can I do to help myself?' This can be the point at which people lose interest. We have become, sadly, a quick fix society and we sometimes find it hard to take responsibility for anything. We prefer to find something or someone outside of ourselves to blame, for whatever is happening to us. We can be a bit lazy too and expect the doctors to do all the work in fixing the asthma and we would like it done quickly so that it doesn't inconvenience our lives. We also have all sorts of reasons why we can't change the asthma such as not knowing where to start or believing it is hereditary which means having to live with it. What about "I'm too old to change now" or "that sounds like too much hard work." Maybe they aren't reasons in so much as they are excuses so as to avoid having to do anything. After all, it is our body, we live with it, day in, day out, so who better to know what would heal it than us.

In my case, it was the medical profession that initially saved my life and for that I can never thank them enough. Without those life-saving drugs and knowledgeable specialists I would not be here today. However, I actually started finding my answers for changing my condition when I looked into the concept of healing the whole body; not just the physical.

What is the whole body?

The whole body encompasses the physical, mental/emotional and spiritual. The spiritual is not connected to anything religious; it is simply your essence, the core self of who you are and it connects us with the Universal Source of All That Is.

To have optimal health these 4 bodies are balanced evenly. In most of us, there is an imbalance. We are often stronger in some areas, weaker in others. When I came across this information I had to really think about how this related to me and it was easy to figure out that the physical body was one of my strongest because of my lifetime of playing sport, working out at the gym and participation in anything related to physical activity, done to almost obsessive levels at times. Another imbalance which took me longer to figure out because it wasn't immediately obvious was that my body wasn't really comfortable being in this world in the first place.

The mental area was another level where I was able to see I may be out of balance; in other words I lived in my head too much. I was constantly thinking and analyzing to the nth degree and was very rigid in my judgement of myself and others.

Looking back now, I can see that I was what is often referred to as a "control freak."

When I thought about the emotional body, it was quite different. I knew instinctively that this area varied a lot from the first two and was not nearly as strong.

I was rarely in touch with my feelings and those I did experience were negative. One emotion that I did outwardly express was anger and when it actually came out I would try and cap it immediately. I was told repeatedly that no-one liked people who couldn't control their temper. Any positive emotion I showed was mild at best because I really wasn't comfortable allowing myself to be too excited or to express great joy.

The spiritual was also low key in that I was brought up with a religious background but was not comfortable with all the rules and belief systems that seemed to be such a big part of all the religions and so was sort of suspended between the outward ideals which didn't quite line up with what I was feeling on the inside. I had always believed in the power of prayer and its use was still very much a part of my life as well as meditation every once in a while. However, I was able to see that although the spiritual body didn't seem to be as suppressed as the emotional body, it was not as strong as the physical and the mental bodies.

If you decide to check out your own different bodies it may be obvious to you right away which ones are stronger or perhaps you may even decide that they are all balanced. From what I read about this particular idea, if there is an illness, then there is most often an imbalance of some kind happening somewhere in those four bodies.

Our physical body is our home while our soul has its experience here and neglecting that body can also be a factor for imbalance. Our eating, drinking and sleeping habits are directly connected to our body and incorrect fueling can lead to an imbalance, if not sooner, then perhaps later. Sometimes it helps also, to check and see if one actually feels comfortable in the body. It may be because of feeling like that for so long, it is not even a conscious awareness any more. Connecting with other human beings by touch is also very important to our well-being and an imbalance may show up if hugging someone or being hugged makes one feel uncomfortable.

From there it is on to the mental body. The same thing goes for thinking. There may be a mind-set where definite ideas of what is right and wrong are very strong in regards to others as well as oneself. There can also be frustration with anyone who disagrees with our opinions on things as well as a need to try and change a person's view to line up with our own. Have a look and see if the mind is flexible in its thoughts or whether it has become rigid and closed.

After the mental we go to the emotional body as these two are tied closely together. First we have the thought and then we attach a feeling to it and more often than not, it is a negative feeling which can be harmful to the body and results in illness when the body reaches its limit of absorption. Check in to see which emotions may be suppressed. Fear, anger, jealousy and guilt are just a few emotions to consider and almost everyone has a fear of 'something', no matter how small. Fear is simply a "Fantasized Experience About Reality" or else "False Evidence Appearing Real". Have an honest look to discover what is hidden inside and how much of an impact it is having on daily life.

Then there is the spiritual and although many feel you cannot be too spiritual, there may be a tendency for it to become a total focus to the exclusion of everything else in life that also needs attention so this may cause an imbalance.

If you are unsure of where the imbalances may be for you, perhaps discussing it with family and friends might be helpful. They often see things and us as we can never see ourselves. A good friend told me many years ago about my strong mental body; about how I was such a deep thinker; it was very obvious to others who knew me and yet I didn't really see that until I started on my own journey.

After working out the areas where the imbalances were, I decided that the mental body was the place to start because until I was ready to look at the way I thought about asthma, it would be hard to make any kind of change. At least, that was the conclusion I came to at the time and it turned out to be the right decision for me.

When I started my search, the first thing I did was let go of all preconceived ideas I had around asthma and approached everything with an open mind. I looked at all possibilities, even if I wasn't able to accept them in that moment. When you are told the same things over and over, sometimes for years, it can become part of your belief system. It may be a big step to look at how we think and why we think as we do and an even bigger step to make a decision to perhaps change the way we think.

We also know that when new discoveries are made, it is often because someone, instead of walking the same old path, has branched out onto a new path, which means going outside the old boundaries. Therefore, it is quite natural if you find yourself feeling resistance about some of the concepts presented in this book. That can be a good sign. It may be because your thinking is being challenged. Sometimes I had resistance or outright denial but also realized that when this happened I needed to pay attention; perhaps here was an opportunity for change; the choice was mine.

Life is full of choices and when it came to my thinking I made the decision to make whatever changes were necessary, both in my conscious and subconscious minds. I realized, through my research, that the subconscious mind was even more powerful than the conscious mind and that was where everything I had experienced in my life up to that point, was stored. To get any results I needed to harness the wisdom in the subconscious mind and make it work for me instead of against me.

If this book has found its way to you, you may be ready for change or there is the potential for change and so I salute you. By relating my journey, all the avenues explored, as well as my successes, I hope to encourage you to orchestrate your own journey and see where it takes you.

NOTE: If you decide to try new techniques, keep your doctor informed and always stay on your medication. There are many doctors who will work with their patients in 'all' aspects of healing because their goal is a healthy patient and they are open to 'change' themselves. Any successful journey is dependent on having a travelling companion that is in accordance with you.

Chapter 3

THE MENTAL BODY

After asthma attacks were no longer a part of my life and I mentioned to people that I had reversed the ailment, they were understandably sceptic. I would often get comments like, "Oh that's because it was just emotional or "it must have been psychological" or "it was just psychosomatic." In actual fact, it wasn't just 'one' thing. It was a holistic approach, addressing the spiritual, mental, emotional and physical body that gave me results.

Today it seems that we are no closer to finding a cure for asthma than we were years ago and I wonder if we need to approach the illness from another direction. Our medications are more sophisticated, the doctors are more knowledgeable and we have many more resources to help us. Instead of starting outside with the physical and going inside, how would it be if we were to start on the inside and work outwards? In holistic medicine it is believed that the physical signs are actually the last sign of illness. By the time we become physically ill, there has been an imbalance in the body for quite some time. It could be in any, all or some of the four bodies but as we are constantly creating our life according to our thoughts, the mental body is a good place to start. Treat that level first, on the

13

inside and eventually results may show up, on the outside, in the physical. Is it time we started looking for the cause as well as using medication?

What is the cause?

As a child in rural Australia the cause was thought to be dust, animal dander, pollen, food allergies, perfume, grass, weather changes etc., Today we know they are all symptoms or triggers; the body's way of telling us it needs healing? What if the cause is on the inside and that is where we can find the answers?

We have created this illness for some reason and we are the ones who can reverse it.

Did you get annoyed reading that last statement? I sure did the first time I came across it. The idea that I would create something that would make my life so miserable was ridiculous. The only reason I had asthma (or so I had always been told and I had no reason to think otherwise) was because my paternal grandmother had been an asthmatic and it was hereditary.

It was a gradual process to realize there was a whole lot more to it than the hereditary factor. Today I realize that in having the genes of my ancestors the wiring was there for asthma but without certain thought patterns, created through my early life experiences, it may not have surfaced at all in my life.

In one of the many articles that I came across on my journey towards wellness, it was written that asthma is known as the 'holding disease'. Apparently, asthmatics can be quite rigid in their thinking (and I had realized right from the beginning that I was such a person) believing that they have to 'hold on', to control the situation to survive.

Having suffered through many scary asthma attacks I know that statement is very true. However, in some cases that need to hold on and to control spills over to our everyday life and is not just during the asthma attacks; hence the rigid thinking. Some asthmatics may not have a problem breathing in; it is in letting the breath go i.e., exhaling, that can also be a problem.

This again may be why it is so hard to think about asthma in any other way than what you have been used to; it can be set in our minds to only think a certain way. If you see yourself this way, there are ways to open up the thinking. There are some good personal development books on the market about learning to 'let go', which is a good way to open the mind up to seeing things in a new or different way and the internet is also a great tool when trying to access new information.

As I look back now I can see, although I was not aware of it at the time, that as soon as I decided to find answers for the asthma, they came along as I was ready for them. The first came in the form of a book, from my father-in-law, who thought I might find it interesting. It was called 'The Power of the Subconscious Mind' by Joseph Murphy. It immediately resonated with me and I started paying attention to my thoughts. From there I went to experimenting with positive affirmations, both written and on tapes. Finally I started recording the affirmations using my own voice as I had heard that one's own voice is very effective in healing oneself.

During this time I did get results with some of my affirmations which was very exciting. However, I did not have any kind of change around the asthma. It was still there and I felt as if I was missing something; somehow the dots did not quite connect.

Then I came upon "You Can Heal Your Life" by Louise Hay. This book had a profound effect upon me. It was about metaphysical healing; still healing the whole body but it went further in linking certain thought patterns to specific illnesses in areas of the body. This made sense to me and made me realize that I needed to discover the thought patterns that were connected to the asthma and discover where they had originated.

In this book listed under asthma in children (which I had been when the attacks started) I found the probable cause to be around not wanting to be alive.

This did not make any sense to me at all at that time as consciously I was quite happy being alive. Admittedly, I had never felt 'at home' here on earth or felt that I belonged here, but that was something different again. At any rate, I was open to the idea of there being some thought, or thoughts, on the subconscious level, that I did not even know existed.

Our brain is a very efficient computer but like all computers it can only work with the information we put into it. That is why it is important to be aware of what we are thinking. The subconscious plays such a big part in our thinking process. Everything we have ever felt, thought, learned or seen, from birth until the present day, is stored there and it is the subconscious that runs our lives most of the time.

Unfortunately, the subconscious does not reason or rationalize and cannot tell if certain thoughts are harmful to the body. It takes everything that comes in, as truth. We are the sum of all our thoughts; the good and the not so good. In order to do something about the asthma, it is necessary to look at the way we think, both consciously and subconsciously.

Our thought patterns have been with us for a long time. They start as soon as we are born and it can be even earlier, in the womb, as I discovered when I started my journey. Then we go to school and are absolute sponges, taking in everything and during the teenage years we add more. In fact, we are continually absorbing and creating thought patterns without realizing it. Each time we see billboards as we are driving we can absorb the message as our brain registers what we see. We watch TV and are continually exposed to advertisements which we register on some level. Perhaps you have the radio on while driving in the car; another way to absorb without realizing it.

Eventually we find ourselves with habitual thought patterns that are contrary to our very essence as a human being because we have been conditioned to think in a particular way. In fact, we may not even be aware that some of our thoughts are not good for us because we have lived with them for so long that they seem natural to us. There is one field of thought which believes that the first seven years of our lives are when we absorb all the main thought patterns that will dictate how we respond to the world around us and how it pertains to us because we cannot differentiate until we reach that age.

Now, if any of these habitual thoughts we have taken on for ourselves are of the type that are harmful to our health, they can gradually cause an imbalance in the body. When that situation becomes too much for the body it often tries to get our attention by manifesting a physical ailment in the hope that we will do something to correct the imbalance our body is feeling. This is the point where the cause needs to be addressed but we have become very adept at doing whatever we can to suppress the symptoms so that we can get on with our lives.

There are a few simple steps we can take towards changing our thinking or at least getting it to look at asthma from a different perspective. These are simple exercises but remember that we have been used to thinking a certain way in regards to asthma.

You may or may not have already noticed that every time you read the word asthma in this book, it will always begin with a small 'a', even if it's the first word in the sentence.

asthma

Notice how this somehow changes the word, how it loses some of its power. This is the start of retraining ourselves to think of asthma as being something that can be overcome. Continuing along these same lines, start changing the way you speak about asthma.

For instance, someone says to you... "How is your asthma today?"

You reply... "My asthma is much better."

Change your reply to... "The asthma is much better,"

In the first instance the speaker is projecting the asthma onto you as if it's something you own and your reply suggests you think you do too. By saying 'the', you stop owning it and you start thinking about it subjectively, putting distance between you and it.

This may not seem like much and may feel a bit silly but every change you make, however small, is another step towards viewing the illness (or any illness for that matter) with a different perspective. Remember...as we think, so we are! When we are impatient and desire all the answers right now, we are plugging into the old programming. The new programming is a desire to learn how the asthma was created and taking steps towards discovery, absorbing any learning we encounter along the way.

There is a connection from the mind to the body in asthma and that is with our lungs and our breathing. Lungs represent Life and asthma cuts off our life force.

Why would we do that to ourselves? Well, consciously, we don't but this is where the subconscious comes in. It has been faithfully storing all thoughts that have come in since birth, some of which could be the activators for the asthma and they keep playing continuously because we don't change them.

Why don't we change those thoughts?

It may be that we are not even aware asthma has any connection to our thoughts or if we do have some idea that there is a connection, we still don't know how to make changes. Perhaps we think that we cannot heal ourselves; that it has to come from someone or something outside of ourselves and then there is the idea that we just have to accept things the way they are and it's no good trying to change anything.

Each one of us is an incredible human being with the capacity to heal ourselves and we can have help to do this in the form of the medical field as well as holistic, metaphysical or alternative medicine (whatever you prefer to call it). Going inside ourselves to start looking for answers is perhaps preferable to giving away our power and expecting others to always do that for us.

Another useful thing to do is question what you actually believe where asthma is concerned. This is something I did at the beginning of my search. I looked at the fact that my grandmother was asthmatic but my brother wasn't so why was it just me? Then there was the 'asthma is incurable' mantra and this was one I never really agreed with but when you are a child you do not argue with adults over some things.

I was constantly told asthma was something I had to learn to live with. This belief was ingrained in me for quite a long time because, as a child, I actually thought I was lucky that my asthma attacks weren't the type that happened all the time. I sometimes had two or three weeks in between attacks so I really did believe that I was fortunate. I knew other asthmatics who had very limited lives because of the frequency of their attacks and they always looked ill, even when not having an attack and I was always the picture of health. I also never caught a cold or had any other kind of lung complaint which was also very different for someone with that condition. Easy to see why my thoughts accepted this idea of learning to live with it, even though it was a very limited way of thinking.

Those were some of my beliefs and you may have different ones but the important thing to ask yourself is if they are really what you believe or were they projected on to you and you just went along with them.

Take some time to create a list of your beliefs, going back to it from time to time as more thoughts come to you. It may take a while to pull everything up from the subconscious and you might, quite possibly, not even be aware you have any beliefs because of being on automatic pilot for so long. For instance: were you told that you were just having the attacks to gain attention or perhaps it was to do with your career; being told there were certain jobs you could never aspire to because of your 'condition'.

After you have made the list, go through each statement and try to remember where they came from and if you do believe them and why. From there you might ask yourself which ones don't really resonate with you, and if that is the case, is there any reason to hang on to them. The mind is very powerful but we are the ones in charge; we can create change.

Chapter 4

THE EMOTIONAL BODY

Once we have opened our thought processes, the next step is to look at the emotional body. The emotions and thoughts are tied together because our thoughts create an emotional reaction in our body no matter what kind of thought we have.

Sometimes we think we have dealt with upsetting events in our lives and don't realize that all we've done is 'think' our way through the experience. We analyze it, compartmentalize it and move on, believing we've done all that needs to be done.

Thinking things through is very good but it is also important to acknowledge the emotional component as well, allowing ourselves to feel the particular emotion that is connected to that thought. We are 'feeling' beings but in some instances we realized that it wasn't always acceptable to express our feelings. At other times, we just didn't know how to express what we were feeling. So, we became very good at hiding them, disguising them, stuffing them deep inside and generally not acknowledging them.

We started this process of suppression for our own protection. It worked for us and so we've kept right on doing it but we are not machines and eventually all that suppression has to come out somehow; quite often as illness. By addressing the emotion we can look at releasing it. Most of us do not know how to do this or even think it is necessary, as it's something we have never been taught to do. There have been times when we've actually been encouraged to not deal with our emotions because it makes those around us feel uncomfortable. I read somewhere that nobody ever died from any illness called 'feeling', but people die every day from illnesses generated by not feeling.

How do we recognize our emotional wounds?

We do that through the people with whom we interact. These people are like teachers for us and they include our family, spouses, our bosses, the co-workers and even our children who can often be our best teachers and we don't see it, mainly because they are children and as such our perception is that we are their teachers.

Sadness, fear, panic, guilt, shame and anger are just some of the emotions we can experience from the time we are born and how we react to them or how they are dealt with at that time, makes a huge difference to our inner well-being.

We would be much healthier and for sure happier, if we learnt to recognize and deal with our emotion 'in the moment' and to then move through it, a wiser and stronger person. When we pretend we are not angry or hurt, we actually do hurt ourselves. As we are not taught how to deal with emotion, it tends to be a largely ignored part of us and our earliest experiences around emotions is with our parents who are not always very good themselves at expressing emotion depending on how their own emotional upbringing was handled. Unless we recognize and are willing to make changes, we will keep doing it the same way in each subsequent generation.

There are many ways to release emotions. Crying is often helpful; some say laughing is very beneficial too. Then there is physical activity, walking, throwing cushions against the wall, punching a pillow or sitting in the car with the windows up while you scream. Sometimes, when one feels the need to cry but for some reason just cannot do so, a sad movie will help. Then, when the tears come, there will be a release that you recognize is not actually a result of watching the movie; it is just a trigger for you to release the emotion bottled up inside. These are just a few ideas that can be helpful for emotional release.

What is important to remember is that we alone are responsible for our emotions. If or when we react to what others say or do, it is because that particular emotion is tied to a subconscious mental pattern we are running and they simply trigger it.

When working on uncovering the emotional wounds, we need to be gentle with ourselves and take however long is needed to move through the process as there may be many layers to address and above all, we need to have compassion for ourselves.

Why is compassion for ourselves important?

Compassion for the self is how we open the door to loving ourselves and if we are experiencing an illness we've fallen out of love with ourselves. Most of us are aware we need to have compassion for others but the second part of that teaching about also applying it to ourselves never happened.

Having compassion for the self is all about seeing and feeling the pain without trying to hide it or fix it; it means looking at it; warts and all, as the saying goes. Once we befriend ourselves the door will open to understanding the "whys" of the illness and steps can be taken towards healing the inner pain.

Loving ourselves and forgiveness of selves is all tied in with our emotions and is a huge part of the healing process. Once we take responsibility for our emotion and then realize that our reactions have been a result of others triggering our suppressed emotions, we can begin to accept ourselves knowing that as we are a work in progress, we are capable of changing.

To create change we must take action. Attending talks, seminars, reading books and watching videos are all good tools to help us change but they can become an intellectual exercise (mental) where we fool ourselves into thinking we are moving forward but in reality we are only going round and round in circles. To implement the learning we need to take action. The subconscious understands action and responds.

Feelings are a natural part of us, like our thoughts. When we decide they are wrong or not acceptable we use a lot of energy to suppress that uncomfortable sensation in our body. I came across a statement once that stated we use 10 times more energy to suppress a feeling than we do to deal with it in the moment. If that is true we are not really using our energy in an optimal way, but rather wasting that precious source which we might use in much more useful ways.

One of the biggest drawbacks to our development are the core beliefs that we are bad, we've done something wrong or we aren't good enough. These beliefs probably weren't meant to cause the pain they did when parents said them. It's just that when we are children, we are very sensitive and wide open, accepting any seeds thrown our way. Through continual planting of these same seeds, good and not so good, a pattern is established and becomes the creed that the child lives by on a daily basis. On top of that comes the conditioning about not letting that emotion out because it often triggers the parents own unhealed wounds which makes them feel uncomfortable.

It is not a fault of anyone as to how this happens, it just does. It is part of the process of where we are now in our human development. A hundred years from now it may be so much better (or we hope so anyway) as we will have learnt so much more, made improvements with each successive generation and learnt that emotions are something to enjoy; not something to use as body stuffing.

When or if you decide to take an interest in making changes or discoveries around asthma, it is good to have this background on thoughts and connection to feelings explained as all healing begins to start when people change their minds and start thinking for themselves with thoughts that resonate or 'feel right' for them.

As thought and emotions are so closely entwined, we can change our emotion (or feeling) when we decide to change our thoughts. If a thought is attached to a specific emotion, that emotion will surface whenever we have the thought. Try this exercise for yourself. Think of a situation or experience you've had in the past that was impactful for you and notice the emotion that surfaces right after the thought. This is happening continually and it is just so automatic that we don't notice or question it.

Once we understand the correlation between the mental/emotional bodies we can create changes that will ensure the emotions that follow our thoughts are more 'in line' with our essence and better health may well be the result.

Chapter 5

FAMILY HISTORY/GENETICS

After delving into the mental and emotional aspect of asthma and becoming more aware of my thinking as well as how my emotions played their part, I knew I needed more information so I looked at my genetics. We know that many ailments seem to get passed down through each generation. As my paternal grandmother had been an asthmatic I made this my starting point to see how long the ailment had been a part of the family ancestry.

Right away I came across some information about certain scientists who had been doing years of research and their findings led them to believe that we needed to go back seven generations before we would be able to determine that a specific ailment was not part of the family genes. If that is the case, people who suddenly start having asthma attacks without any history or knowledge of it in their immediate family, may be unknowingly inheriting genes from previous ancestors which are being triggered in this generation. After all, how many families can go back that far in their history and if they do, many times it is only names and dates they have – not details on the actual people's lives.

In some families, one or two members may have the

inherited illness while one or two may not. How does that happen? They all have the same genetics. There may be several reasons but consider the 'thought pattern'. The genetics or 'wiring' is there in all four people but perhaps it is the inherited 'thought' pattern that activates it and as we all think differently, there's a good chance our path in life will be different as well. I'm not saying that the solution is that black and white but it is just another aspect to consider to be open to 'thinking' about, as we go looking for answers on our journey.

By the time I decided to go looking for answers in my family history, a lot of the people who could have helped me in my quest were already deceased. All I was able to discover was that my paternal grandmother (who died before I was born) had asthma all her life; it started when she was a child. There didn't seem to be any evidence of it with any of her siblings but by researching what little pieces I could find of their lives, I was able to put together a picture of sorts. My paternal Great Grandmother was not an asthmatic but that was as far as I could go with finding out any more information.

My Dad was a great help in telling me all he remembered about his aunts and uncles and from the time I was quite little I had been told many times that asthma always came out in every other generation. Whether this is true or not is a moot point. I just know that Dad and his siblings did not have asthma, but here I was, the next generation and I did have it, so on that subconscious level, I accepted that thought pattern even though I was not aware of doing so at the time.

My father remembered his mother having attacks all his life. They lasted a few hours and at times were very severe. The remedy used in those days was an asthma powder, burnt on the lid of a tin and the fumes inhaled like a vaporizer.

Thinking about a thought pattern that may have started my

grandmother's life of asthma, I went through what I knew of her life. One thing I found is that her father died when she was eight years of age.

When I was researching every avenue for causes of asthma I did come up with some reasons that were considered a possibility as a trigger for the onset of asthma.

They are…

… being abandoned

… experiencing a loss

… holding grief inside and not being able to let it out

I don't know how old my grandmother was as a child when the asthma started; whether she had it before her father died or whether it came on as a result of the trauma of losing him.

As an interesting aside, in my own case, although the asthma started at a much younger age, it took a drastic turn to become more debilitating when I was eight. At that time my neighbor, who was like a surrogate grandpa and whom I adored, died suddenly of a heart attack. I had a very severe attack of asthma on the day of his funeral and could not attend the service. This was a devastating loss for me and I did feel abandoned and lost without him for a very long time.

It was an interesting fact to discover that both my grandmother and I, who were both asthmatics, also had the same experience of losing a loved one at the same age.

Whether it had any effect on my grandmother's condition or if it was the start of it, I will never know but it certainly does open the door to speculation.

Finding out as much as you can about the family history and what part asthma plays in it with other relatives is just one more way of opening up the mind to a broader view of things. After all, life is not always black or white; there are many shades of grey.

While it may not always be possible to have precise facts to back up suppositions it is the opening up of possibilities to us that is important. Life isn't an exact science. How can it be when those living it are feeling beings, not machines? And it is important to remember too, that this is simply my story; my discoveries and how I related them to me and my condition. However fanciful they may seem to you, they provided answers to me and helped me learn more about what part asthma played in my lineage.

Chapter 6

MY LIFE WITH aSTHMA

asthma affects everyone differently, from the things that trigger an attack, to the severity of an attack, to how long it lasts and how often one happens. Because of that fact it is probably best at this time to tell you my history with the asthma, up to the point where I went into the coma. You will then have a good point of reference as well as an understanding when you read the different techniques I tried and the discoveries I made before the coma and then after the coma as well.

My problems began at birth. I was a transverse lie, (sideways in the womb), the birth involved forceps and once born I almost died because the doctor had a lot of difficulty trying to get me to take that all important first breath.

According to my parents (plus the information written in my baby book) I had my first attack at five years of age and it occurred when I was told I would have to wait until I was six to go to school. Apparently this was a terrible disappointment for me. After that initial attack, they happened randomly and lasted for as long as it took for the medication to take affect; usually a few hours.

I do remember that before I started taking any kind of medication, mum used to make mustard plasters for my attacks which I would wear against my chest and back with a tight vest over the top to hold it in place. This was used at night time, to facilitate easier breathing as well as helping me to sleep. Many years ago this was a remedy that was widely used to help with chest and lung congestion. I have no idea if it ever did the trick; all I remember is going to bed feeling funny because it felt like I was still dressed.

Soon after the asthma began I was tested for allergens and it was discovered I had a reaction to dust, grasses, feathers, all fur bearing animals, and pollens. These triggers set off the hay fever which usually continued until it developed into an asthma attack. I also had another trigger which was a bit different. As we lived in the country it was very exciting, as a child, to go to the city for the day. However, my mother could never tell me beforehand if we were going because I would wake up with asthma and be unable to go.

Being woken up that morning, being told we were off to the city and getting ready to do so, somehow prevented the attack. I do not know if there were other instances where this technique was used by my mother to avoid an attack but I remember her telling me of this one when I was older.

Around the age of fourteen I started having an all-day hay fever attack that always occurred on a Sunday and was exhausting, resulting in my mouth breaking out in fever blisters on the Monday.

Both my parents were smokers, from the time I was quite young onwards. As smoke was not something that came up in the allergens testing, I'm sure it never occurred to them, or was even suggested, that they give it up because it might be detrimental to my health. As it was, they made many changes, in and around the house, to help with my condition.

When I was eight years old, a new kind of attack began

occurring. This one lasted for a whole week and it was always the same. I would wake up with asthma on a Monday morning and gradually the intensity of the attack would increase as the week progressed until Saturday. In the afternoon on that day it would begin to subside and by Sunday it was gone. However, on that day I was often quite tired after a week of fighting to breathe and there was also a lot of pain in my back (at that time it was explained to me that this was due to the lungs subsiding back to their original size, having been over expanded for a prolonged time during the attack).

From then on I had two types of attacks happening. The one kind could be stopped with medication (tablets) and they occurred at any time. The week long attack could not be stopped and always ran from Monday to Saturday. No amount of tablets had any affect and an injection (the only alternative at that time) just took the edge off the attack, enabling me to cope until it ran its course. These injections were not a common occurrence. In fact, they were few and far between because it was feared I would build up an immunity to them and then they would not work anymore.

How often I had these week long episodes had no rhyme or reason either as sometimes they would be a month apart or maybe five or six weeks; many times I would only have a week free and back it would come again. At that time, one didn't go to the hospital; the doctor came to the house if it was necessary. There were many times when I was terrified that I was going to die and begged for an injection, only to have it refused because I'd had one only three weeks before. Looking back now I wonder how I made it through some of those attacks but we humans are quite resilient at times.

Sleeping was almost impossible during the week long attacks. When I was young I would spend my nights kneeling in bed, resting my forehead on my hands as that seemed to be the only way I could get relief. As I became older I found it easier to sit up all night in the living room, leaning forward in the chair and resting my head on my folded arms on a table. It gave me some relief but very little sleep. Sometimes I would become very scared on the Friday nights, which was when the attack seemed to reach its peak and I found that distracting my mind was the only way I could cope so I used to count, first by twos, then fours, then sixes and so on, until I calmed myself down.

You might think that I did not have much of a life with all these attacks but it was really quite normal and I just learned to live with asthma as a part of my life. When the asthma first started it was not something new for my dad; he had grown up with this ailment in the family. However, my mum had no knowledge of it at all and was happy to be guided as to what to do, to help me. The doctor thought the attacks were my way of trying to get attention so it was decided I wasn't to be pampered or catered to when they occurred. The thinking was that if I didn't get the desired reaction I would stop having them. My parents followed these instructions faithfully for years but still the attacks continued to occur.

It was also advised that I take part in sport, especially swimming, to develop my lung capacity. As we lived inland with no swimming facilities, I instead participated in all the sports offered at school as well as joining the local Netball and Tennis clubs.

Fortunately I was athletic and loved sport so this set the pattern for my whole life; a life of fitness.

Staying home from school during every week long attack was not a regular occurrence (due to the theory of my just wanting attention) so I would go off to school, just up the road and it would take forever to get there. I could only walk a few steps and then would have to sit and get my breath. I do remember days that were so bad that I had to stay home. Attending school during an attack was very hard; all my concentration and energy was on breathing so trying to do the schoolwork as well was a bit of a struggle.

I attended a private school and Sports Day was on a Saturday afternoon in the elementary grades so the parents could attend. I was always hoping I wouldn't have one of my week long episodes around that time as I was sports mad and very competitive. I only remember one occasion quite vividly where I had been ill all week but I was determined to compete. Being a Saturday, the attack was starting to subside by the afternoon and I convinced my mum that I was actually better than I was. I ran in all the races and took part in the team events as well and in between I was in the bathroom vomiting; looking back I am probably lucky I didn't have worse reactions. Our team won the trophy that day so it was all worth it to me. I do remember my mum saying I was never going to be allowed to do that again.

This state of affairs with two types of attacks happening continued until I was fifteen. At that time a 'puffer' came onto the market for asthma and it worked like a charm for stopping the short attacks; to me this was a miracle. One spray of the puffer and I was back to normal breathing; no more sitting quietly waiting for the pills to take effect. The week long attacks stopped by themselves around this time too and that coincided with my starting to go out to work. As I'd always been told the asthma might go away when I 'grew up' I presumed this was what had happened.

About three years later I moved to the city to work and the asthma and hay fever stopped altogether. I also took up smoking, as an act of defiance I think, because I was tired of people always telling me smoking was something I could never do because of being an asthmatic. However, for the few years that I did indulge in the habit, it was always in a part time capacity. I controlled it; it never controlled me and I had no trouble quitting.

I married a Canadian in 1970 and in 1971 my husband and I moved to Vancouver, Canada to live. Although I had not had any asthma for several years I still carried a puffer, replacing it as it expired. I'd had the same brand since I began using them at age fifteen. I discovered in Canada that my brand had been pulled from the market quite some time before because it was found that prolonged use may cause heart attacks.

About two years after moving to Canada, the attacks came back; they had been gone for approximately seven years. It was a bit of a surprise to have this happen. I had been told that often, when you have asthma as a child, it can come back again when you get older but I expected that meant when I was elderly; not when I was in my twenties. I had known a lady in that exact situation when I was growing up and she was in her late seventies at the time. For the most part, each attack I had was exercise induced and once again, one spray of the puffer would take it away. The allergies also came back, along with the day-long sneezing attacks on Sundays.

We decided to start a family and several months before we did I gave up smoking and the asthma disappeared altogether so I didn't have the worry of wondering how my taking medication would affect our baby. About six months after our son was born the asthma re-appeared in the same format as before, as a result of exercise or strenuous exertion. I took up part time smoking again when our son was two and a half.

It was around this time that I really started thinking about asthma and ways to do something about it and that is when information and different avenues to get information started to appear in my life. It was a slow process as life and family took precedence over everything. Looking for answers was something that felt more like a hobby at times; something I would get to when I had some spare time. I was anxious to make headway with my search but at times life had a way of taking over and I was sidetracked and distracted.

I had continued to be physically active in my life up to this point and I began playing and competing in Netball again, at the Provincial and National level and my fitness level was at an all-time high. At this point I gave up smoking forever and the asthma was never a problem. Occasionally I would feel a bit wheezy at the beginning of a workout or during a warm-up session prior to a game but the usual use of the puffer would take it away.

In 1986 I contracted bronchitis. Antibiotics cleared up the condition but a few months later I caught pneumonia and was back on antibiotics. It was now going into the Christmas season, Netball was shutting down until the New Year and then my father in law suddenly passed away and things were very chaotic through that time. As I was feeling much better by this time I sort of relegated my state of health to the back burner to deal with the immediate family tragedy. When January came round, I thought I was completely recovered and so returned to Netball. However, I found I could hardly breathe; something was very wrong. My doctor confirmed that I had a lung infection as the pneumonia had not really cleared up and so it was arranged for me to see a specialist.

It needs to be said at this time that I was at fault in this instance for not going back to the doctor to get the 'all clear' after the second round of antibiotics, due to the family events that occurred and if I had done so the resulting infection may not have happened.

The specialist sent me for x-rays and breathing tests. The results of the breathing test were well below par and when I saw the x-ray and was shown all the areas where there was lung damage, as well as exposure to TB, I was shocked. I knew I had never had TB; when I immigrated here that was one of the strict conditions around being accepted into the country. There was to be no evidence of TB or exposure to it either and I had passed all those tests. (I still wonder, to this day, if those x-rays were really mine).

At that time I was put on two different puffers, one a steroid, four times a day and told that my life, as I knew it, was over. I'd never play sports again and could consider myself lucky if I even had the capacity to do vacuuming and I would be on medication for the rest of my life. At this point I think I went into shock.

I absolutely refused to accept the diagnosis but did agree to take the medications that were prescribed. I informed the specialist that when I came to see him in six months (he wanted me there in four) I would be in good health, once again playing Netball and with the help of my family doctor, be able to cut back on the medications.

My family doctor (of ten years) was actually quite shocked at this sudden decline in my health. I was extremely fit because of competing in Netball at the International level and I was in very good health. This resulting condition just did not add up. She suggested that I take a look at my life; to see if there was a possibility something could be triggering this sudden condition.

I had to take drastic measures to recover so I stepped down from the National Netball team. (Canada was going to Scotland to compete in the World Championships in four months) and stopped playing the sport altogether and rested the lungs to allow them to recover from the infection.

By the time I went to see the specialist after six months, I was playing Netball again, at league level, was off all the added medication and just needed the puffer every now and again. I was advised to return to see him if my condition deteriorated.

Everything was good for about eighteen months and then in 1989 I noticed that the asthma was starting to increase again. I had returned to the work force after a nine year absence and some mornings I would wake up quite wheezy but it would subside as soon as I arrived at work. I was also having to use the puffer more often when playing Netball. At other times I would start to wheeze and yet there didn't seem to be a reason for it. However, the puffer would still work in those instances.

Then things started going downhill. I was having attacks that would not go away with the use of the puffer. About two or three times in a span of about nine months I had to go to the emergency department at the hospital to get help with the attack. After a few hours there for treatment I was able to return home and would be okay the next day. As it was getting harder to play Netball I decided to take the last half of the season off. I also resigned from my job and I was starting to feel a bit desperate at this point, not knowing what to do next but knowing something had to be done as I could not go on like this.

I was due to attend the BC Winter Games in Penticton as an Official Umpire for Netball in the February and I was able to participate in that but I knew I wasn't doing well as any kind of real exercise was getting to be very difficult and I was using the puffer constantly. I still believed though, that with rest, it would eventually improve. Several weeks after that I woke up on a Monday morning with an asthma attack in progress. As it had been so many years since those week long attacks I'd had as a child, I did not recognize what was happening and all my husband knew was that I'd had asthma as a child so he had no real information to give to the medical staff at the hospital either and whether that would have even made any difference is something we'll never know. By Tuesday morning I was in very bad shape; breathing was almost impossible and the puffer was having no effect whatsoever; I knew I was in trouble. When my husband arrived home from work that night we went to the emergency at the hospital and what happened next you read about in the first chapter.

It was 1990, the 20th of March and my birthday; I turned 42 that day!

Chapter 7

DISCOVERIES BEFORE
THE COMA

This chapter is going to detail every single thing I tried in my quest to discover the inner cause of asthma 'before' I went into the coma. If you have come to a point where you can look at different ideas and treatments for asthma as possibilities to help the condition, this chapter may be of interest to you. Some of the things I tried may seem unbelievable or weird, perhaps too out there and not something you will ever be able to accept and that is okay. Remember, we are all very individual with the freedom to be and do what feels right for us.

However, there may be others who will be interested, excited, and even eager to start their own journey and have been waiting for someone or something to show them how or to just point the way; to get them started, so to speak. Helping each other is a big part of our learning here as we tend to be hermits in that we either 'do' for ourselves or sometimes don't 'do' at all because asking for help may be seen as a sign of weakness when it is actually a sign of strength.

I've given talks to asthma groups and seen various reactions from people such as complete denial, to those who wanted proof that I've done what I say I've done. There were others who were sure nothing would work for them because their asthma was different, along with the disinterested ones who whispered and giggled through most of the presentation.

People will always react according to their comfort zone in any given situation and I understand that; have even done it myself; we are human after all. I found there were usually one or two at those talks who welcomed all the information I could give them; their eyes would light up with excitement and at the end of the night they were keen to chat, to tell me what small steps they thought they may be able to take; to create a change for themselves. My advice was always to make sure they check with their doctor first, about anything new they wanted to try in regards to their treatment

The very first thing I became involved with was Hatha Yoga in Australia and that was when I was a teenager. My reasons for doing it had nothing to do with asthma (I was not having attacks at that time) but was more about relaxation. I did, however, notice a difference in my breathing right away. I was breathing deeper and fuller and I'm sure this was a good thing for the lungs. There was also a spiritual element to this exercise which appealed to me on some level as well. Even though I really enjoyed each session, it wasn't something I kept doing on a regular basis but over the years I have gone back to it numerous times and always notice changes in my breathing while I am attending the classes.

It was many years later, in Vancouver, that I was told about a Regression therapist who was having an 80% success rate working with asthmatics. I knew nothing about Regression or Hypnosis but was open to trying it. The sessions turned out to be the first big breakthrough in my search. The therapist, through working with asthmatics, found that there was

42

usually three instances where breathing was somehow severely restricted. After the third instance a pattern was established, locked in and then constantly triggered

I found this idea fascinating and was only too happy to try it out but didn't think at this point there would be much of a result because I didn't know of any instances where I had suffered any breathing restrictions, apart from the attacks themselves. For some reason I didn't think I could be hypnotized either; mentally I always maintained control. The first surprise was going into that altered state very easily. I was then led backwards, back to before I was even in the womb and at this point I am wondering what on earth is going on as there is nothing to go to. Then I was asked to move forward.

I was amazed that suddenly I saw a scene in my mind's eye which I was asked to describe and then told to move forward and keep describing what I was seeing as I did so.

Very shortly after that directive I saw hands coming around my neck, from behind, and I started struggling to breathe as I continued describing, step by step, all the physical sensations I was experiencing in the body. These included my face becoming really hot as if it was burning, followed by my eyes feeling as though they were bulging out of their sockets. Then came intense pain in my head which was excruciating and it felt like the top of my head was going to explode. Finally something popped into the opening in my throat and it seemed to be about the size of a ping pong ball. The intensity was almost unbearable and then it all suddenly stopped. There was nothing for a minute or so and then I felt a funny feeling, like leaving or floating away or something. When the therapist asked me 'what is happening now', I calmly announced that I was dead. He gradually brought me back to present time and we discussed what was for me, an amazing experience. He told me I had gone through the whole process of strangulation and dying and had described it perfectly. The ping pong ball feeling was from the Adam's apple popping into the throat opening. Before this experience I did not know there was such a thing as past lives but what I went through had to come from somewhere. I knew it wasn't my imagination; I couldn't or wouldn't imagine being murdered and until then I had no idea what the body actually experienced in the different stages of being strangled.

However, it did explain a couple of lifelong fears I'd had since I was a child. One was having people stand behind me in a line-up, especially if they came too close. It made me antsy to have someone look over my shoulder and I always needed everyone to be in front of me where I could see them. In a crowd I was always at the back and being fairly tall, my reasoning was always that shorter people wouldn't be able to see if I was in front of them.

The other fear was walking in the dark, constantly looking behind me, all the while having my mum tell me that as I had already walked back there, I knew there was nothing there and that it was more important to look ahead because I didn't know what was there. It was also hard for me to wear anything tight around my neck. I had to wear a tie for school as part of the uniform and I always made sure it was a bit looser so that there was no constriction. Now all my fears made sense and over the next few months they actually cleared up which was amazing in itself after years of living with them as part of my life.

This was the first breathing restriction event.

In a month or so I went back for another session, not knowing what to expect.

Once again, I went into the altered state easily and was taken backwards again to when I was in the womb. The therapist stopped at two weeks before birth and started counting down…

fourteen days from birth, thirteen days from birth etc. I was quietly sitting and listening, experiencing nothing until the therapist said: six days from birth: Suddenly my whole body went rigid and then I started to squirm and twist and I could feel my face becoming quite hot and I was struggling to breathe and it was unbearable and I could see in my mind's eye that there was this thick thing around my neck and I tried to claw at it to move it. I was in so much distress having this experience that the therapist immediately started the process of gradually bringing me out of the altered state and back to present time.

I came to realize, after discussing it with the therapist, that what I had seen in my mind's eye was the umbilical cord around my neck. I had no first-hand information on anything like that happening before I was born but I was aware there had been problems prior to and during my birth. So here was the second breathing restriction event.

Now we went looking for that all important third instance. In my baby book, which was quite detailed, my mother had written that I was five when the first asthma attack occurred. A few months later I went back to have another session and this time we had no luck at all. I was taken right through that year when I was five years of age and although some lovely memories surfaced, there was nothing to suggest any sort of breathing problem. It was decided that I would contact my dad (mum had already passed away) and ask if we were looking in the right year. I wrote and explained to him what I was doing and asked if he was sure I was five at the onset of the asthma and I was assured it was definitely at that age.

Once again we went into that year trying to discover if there was something that had been missed and still nothing came up; there was no reaction to anything. At this point, there was nothing more that could be done. However, just those two sessions and releasing those trapped emotions had an effect and there was a big improvement in my condition in the months afterwards. I did not need to use the puffer at all. My allergies also cleared up (apart from the Sunday episodes) to the point where we were able to have a cat and a guinea pig in house. Touching fur bearing animals or even just being in the same room with them without touching them had not been possible before those sessions. Now I had no reactions at all and as I love cats it was a joy to walk around holding the cat and not sneeze, nor have my eyes itch and swell or welts come up on my arms from having to scratch as had occurred in the past. As the allergic reactions to the animals would most often lead to wheezing, this also disappeared when the allergies cleared up.

When I contracted the lung infection years later I also took some different steps in my quest to reverse the condition. Quite often I would follow my intuition and that is how I came to book a reading with a well- respected, very reputable Medium. As soon as I sat down she began talking about my lungs and the condition they were in (without me having even opened my mouth at this point) and told me two things that would help. One was visualization. I was to get a picture of lungs, color them pink and put that picture on my fridge where I would see it all the time and visualize my lungs as being that way, pink and healthy.

The second thing was to do breathing exercises from a book called Science of Breath by Yogi Ramacheraka. I was told to read the book and I would know instinctively which exercises I needed to do and I needed to do them twice a day. As I had been working with the power of the mind and visualization for a few years already I knew these things would work. I read the book; there were lots of different breathing exercises and I recognized right away, the ones I was supposed to do.

Another thing I did, which I found from an advertisement

in a magazine, was to order two cassette tapes which had subliminal messages for health programmed into the music. I listened to those tapes every morning and again last thing at night. I had given up running, to allow the lungs to heal but was walking instead and for the whole walk I would also listen to the subliminal message tape. For six months I did all these different things and after just one month I noticed a big difference. I was able to gradually reduce the medication to twice a day and still be free of asthma. Eventually, by the end of the six months, when I went back to playing Netball I was off all the medication once again.

When the asthma started becoming a problem again, eighteen months later, I came across some information that stated Naturopaths had a lot of success with asthmatics so I went that route next and for a few months I was given a lot of different remedies, trying to find that one which would address the problem. It just never happened and it was around this time that I came to a conclusion of my own; that there was some emotional problem that I needed to address; that was where I would find my answers.

This was the last thing I pursued in looking for answers 'before' the coma and by now the asthma was really becoming a problem and I was increasingly frustrated with the whole situation and quite frankly, did not know what to do next or even where to look. I felt mentally exhausted and as this had always been my strong point and I was normally able to fall back on "thinking" up solutions to everything, it was scary for me to suddenly have no clear direction in which to go.

Chapter 8

DISCOVERIES AFTER
THE COMA

It took quite a few months to recover after I came out of the coma and it was seventeen months before I went back into the work force. However, I believe that healing on many levels began the moment I became conscious.

First of all, it is necessary to say that I had been put into an induced coma so that the doctors could try and stop the asthma attack and that every hour, for the duration of the coma, I was given the drug Pavulon, to keep me in that state and machines were helping me to breathe. Pavulon did what it was supposed to do but one of the side effects of the drug is that it atrophies muscles and at that time, being quite fit, I was all muscle and so by the time I came out of the coma I was minus 22 lb. (or 9.979 kg) of that muscle. No muscles meant no ability to move so I was temporarily paralyzed. That state gradually changed as the drug worked its way out of my system and I began the work of strengthening my muscles so that I was able to do the simplest of tasks like feeding myself and walking unaided.

Three weeks out of the coma, when I was starting to feel a little more like me, I went through a very emotional period, which I did not understand at the time. I likened it to opening

Pandora's Box, which, once opened, could not be closed. For a few days I was completely at the mercy of my feelings and was continually running the whole gamut of emotions. I would go from feeling okay to being really happy to being absolutely euphoric and just as quickly come crashing down and feel real despair and that would move into patches of anger and sadness and back into joy again and on and on it went until it ran its course. It was as if all those emotions I had suppressed for years had all been let out at once. I managed to work my way through the whole episode and because of being in such a weakened state, I was amazed I was able to cope with it as it took a couple of days to complete. But along with what was happening was also a thought which kept coming in from somewhere; you never get more than you can handle. Because of that thought I knew somehow I would be okay.

While in the hospital I used affirmations on a daily basis. Being unable to move, there was not a lot I could do physically and my mind was feeling the inactivity so I gave it something to do; each day I would say, over and over to myself, 'tomorrow I will be able to do one more thing than I can do today' and the next day I would spend time looking for that one thing, however small, that showed me I was on the way to recovery. Maybe it would be the slightest of movement in a little finger or a tiny twitch in one of my legs.

As creating what I desired to have in my life had also become a regular exercise since reading Shakti Gawain's, Creative Visualizations many years before, I once again used that system to give myself some focus and direction. I had been told, soon after coming out of the coma, that it would be a long time before I recovered and I may be in hospital for months. Well! This didn't sit well with me at all as that would mean missing out on summer. I was determined that I would not spend one more day in the hospital than was necessary. So I looked to the future and decided that I would be out of the hospital by Mother's Day, which was six weeks away. Everyone humored me by going along with my idea even though privately they thought it was impossible. I couldn't even move; how was I going to be able to walk or even be out of the hospital by then. I started visualizing myself walking into a favorite local Restaurant to have breakfast with my family.

Day in, day out, I held onto that picture in my mind, running through the whole scenario, even down to what I would order to eat and what kind of day it would be. At the same time I also worked very hard on my physical recovery. At first, when I couldn't move at all I had my son, when he came to visit, along with friends, help me do exercises while we visited. They would bend and lift and move my arms and legs for me. So, although others were a bit shocked, it was no surprise to me that I was out of the hospital and home in time to go to the restaurant with my family for Mother's Day and it all unfolded exactly as I had envisioned.

I knew I was getting better on the morning I woke up to an itchy nose, like someone was tickling it with a feather or something and without thinking I automatically lifted my arm to rub my nose. However, with very little muscle control it was like a missile on a deadly path once it started moving and so my arm crashed onto my face with such a force I thought I had broken my nose. Once I got over the shock I was really excited and moved it up and down a few more times to make sure it wasn't a fluke. I was finally making some progress. I also thought it was amazing that in all the time I had been ill and paralyzed I had never had an itch anywhere, prior to that morning.

Once out of the hospital I was still on several types of

medications, to be taken four times a day. It was like I could not even feel my own body and I wondered if I would even realize I was having a problem, if one arose, as the medication seemed to be masking my normal feelings and reactions. This was my take on the whole thing at that time. The only natural healing I did at this time was to take Silica on a regular basis because my skin was as thin as paper due to the steroids I'd taken while in the hospital and my hair was quite thin as a result of most of it falling out after the coma.

About seven weeks out of hospital I flew to Australia to see my father. As I'd seen while out of my body, that he was going to die quite soon, I was anxious to visit with him before that happened and we hadn't seen each other for twelve years. The visit turned out to be very special and I knew, from the moment I arrived and looked into his eyes, that he was ready to leave and had just been waiting for me to come home one last time. It was during this visit that my dad told me I was actually three when the asthma started and not five, as they had led me to believe and he told me the story about it.

The day my baby brother came home from the hospital and I saw him, I freaked out and started screaming and crying for them to take him away, to send him back, I didn't want a brother. Mum and Dad were totally shocked at my reactions as they had prepared me for this event and I had been excited about a new baby. Dad said I could not be consoled and my level of distress was such that I had my first asthma attack, right there and then. Dad said their reasoning for keeping it hidden from me was due to the fact that they both thought I wouldn't have a very good relationship with my brother if I was told how I hadn't wanted him there in the first place. My brother and I were never really close but I put that down to there being three years between us, more than anything else.

My parents sure went to great lengths to cover it all up and if I hadn't almost died from that asthma attack I am not sure I would have ever been told about it.

Over the next few months I gradually lessened the medication until I was off it completely and there was no sign of the asthma at all, even when I did physical exercise. However, I still desired to get to the inner cause; to make sure I wouldn't ever get it again. After I went back to work a co-worker told me about a technique called Rebirthing which had something to do with breathing. I intuitively knew I had to find out more about this process and so went searching. Rebirthing, or Conscious Breathing as it is also called, was developed by Leonard Orr in the 1970's. It is a breathing process which allows us to release emotions that have been suppressed or locked in the body, sometimes since birth and to dissolve what we've held onto for many years and so free up tremendous amounts of life force energy.

I was able to find a person locally who was a Practitioner and went to try it out. It was an hour session during which time I did nothing more than breathe, but the results were amazing as it produced physical reactions in my body that allowed suppressed emotional patterns to surface, often with a picture from the past to go with that emotion, which was then integrated. Over the course of the next couple months I did ten sessions with the Practitioner and during that time I integrated a lot of emotion that was trapped in my body and had realizations around most of it. On some occasions it would be a thought that would pop into my head during the session, to be followed by an emotion and that seemed to trigger the memory or situation that caused the pattern to be locked in originally. It was fascinating how the whole process worked and all from the breathing which made sense as breathing and life go together.

After the ten sessions I was able to do sessions by myself and I did so, every couple of days, for four months. You allow some time in between for the next layer that is ready to be integrated to rise to the surface for processing. I didn't know what I was looking for or why I was doing the sessions so often but I just knew I needed to do so.

This one morning I started the session and within a few minutes I felt my body starting to go quite rigid and then a vibration started inside, like a low hum which I could feel moving up my body from the sacrum area and although this will seem strange, to me it was like a dandelion plant being pulled all the way out, root and all. By the time it got to my throat it erupted as a wailing sound with such a feeling of utter sadness; and I could see myself, in my mind's eye, as a baby. I started to cry and as the tears ran down my face I started to shake uncontrollably and I was sobbing as I started saying over and over, I don't want to be here, I don't want to be here. I allowed my body to integrate the emotion and as my breathing began to regulate once again, I was able to feel a calmness come over me; almost like a relief that I'd finally been able to let go of that pain and agony I'd suppressed for so long.

After the first emotional session I didn't know what to expect at the next one. It started off quite normally and about ten minute into the session I went from warm to being absolutely freezing cold and while trying to breathe through that I heard a man's voice say, 'Mrs. Jones, you have a baby girl' and immediately the thought came into my head. "Johnnie will be so disappointed." I knew instinctively that the thought was coming from my mum and that my dad did not want me because I was a girl. (Right or wrong, that was what I decided, right there and then) It produced such feelings of desolation, sorrow and sadness within me while the adult part of me felt such a wave of compassion for that little baby and what it was experiencing. The breath helped me to integrate that past experience that was locked in my subconscious and this time I was able to see the right of it, how it was part of my journey here and I embraced the knowing I now had; my perception had been changed.

The following session went quite smoothly until about half way through and then I felt a sharp stabbing pain in the base of my skull, like a knife or something jabbing at me. Gradually the pain lengthened, like someone was scraping something down the back of my head and the pain was excruciating. When these sensations arise, the tempo of the breath is changed to accommodate what we are going through and gradually the sensations subside, the body releases its tension and once it has all been integrated, one finishes the session in a state of peace, joy and relaxation. It was after the session that I realized I had been experiencing the forceps, digging at my head, trying to get a grip, to pull me out... it is not a very good feeling for the baby; I felt the pain. The other side of the forceps was attached to the front on my head but during the session there was no pain in this area, just a pressure, like something pushing on the front of my head.

The next several sessions were normal in that I breathed all the way through but nothing dramatic was there although we do process things in every session; it is just that we do not need to have conscious awareness of every single little thing that is in our subconscious. Then came another session where I found my ankles starting to hurt, to the point where it was again very painful and my whole body was smarting; my skin was burning, my back was hurting and I felt very dizzy; everything seemed to be spinning somehow. I was screaming in my head to my mother, 'help me, help me; make it stop' but there was no response from her. I integrated it all, again knowing it was all part of my journey and finding it fascinating that I could actually go back to my birth and know what I had gone through at that time.

Note: Right after I was born the doctor could not get me to take that first breath and my mother did tell me this. She also said that afterwards the nurse said to her, "Mrs. Jones, if you could have seen what the doctor was doing to your baby, to get her to breathe, you would have got up off that table and given him a piece of your mind". She never did tell my mother what it was he was doing but I felt it all; being held by the ankles and hit repeatedly I'd say which would have accounted for the 'smarting' feeling I felt on my skin. The back pain was possibly from suddenly being straightened after nine months of being curved in the womb and the dizzy feeling may have been from being swung around somehow. At any rate, whatever the doctor did obviously worked as I started crying (and according to mum, continued to do so for the next six weeks.)

I had a few sessions where it was a regular breathing session until another layer of the birth trauma presented itself. I started feeling very cold about five minutes after I began and this can be normal as it is the energy moving. However, the feeling of coldness intensified and then the thoughts came that there must be something wrong with me, nobody wants me, I'm all alone. I could get no sense of my mother at all and my body felt tightly contained again but I could breathe okay this time.

Note: Even though I was aware on my adult level what this was all about, I still had to go through it and integrate its rightness. I was told my mother hemorrhaged soon after my birth and she almost died on the table; I can imagine it was a very frantic time for all those concerned.

For a long time after that I cut back on sessions and did them maybe once every two weeks or even less often than that. Sometimes I would do a session if I was aware of something building up in my body as the breathing was wonderful for releasing and relaxing tension. One afternoon, during what I thought would be that type of session I found, as I was breathing, that my shoulders were hunching up past the bottom of my ears and my body was being squeezed and everything was getting very tight. Then my head started to hurt and it kept wanting to turn, to get away from something and I could not breathe. I started making rasping noises in my throat and I needed to loosen something around my neck but my arms were wedged into my sides somehow. It was scary but I knew I was okay; I did live through this; whatever it was and to keep breathing into it. I kept trying to move my head but there didn't seem to be enough room and just when I thought I could not breathe anymore, my head jerked backward and as it did so, I saw a rope like thing slip from under my chin up over my head and I could breathe again. That was an amazing session.

There have been many sessions since that time and I still do them to this day; they are a great way to release stress immediately so that it does not stay in the body and since all those sessions there has been no asthma whatsoever. It would have been more of a statement and proof positive perhaps if all this had happened with a practitioner but it didn't; it was something I had to experience on my own; as I did when it first occurred.

As I'd been looking for the 'root cause' of the asthma all along, I felt I had found it at last. The first session was so symbolic with the pain and hurt rushing up through the body from the sacrum area and having the physical sensations of a root, literally being ripped all the way out.

It was some time after this that I was able to put together what may have been the cause of the week long attacks but because I have no proof it is only supposition. As I was transverse or crossways in the womb my dad told me that my mother had to go into the hospital a week before I was born. At that time they straightened me (the six day reaction in regression perhaps) and bound her so that I could not move back to that crosswise position. As I was born on a Saturday I am guessing that it may have been the Monday when this procedure was done. Knowing from regression and the rebirthing that the cord was around my neck, I would have struggled to breathe for those six days prior to being born. Friday night was always the worse night during my week long attacks; so often I thought I would die. If my mother was already in labor at that time, I would have been in quite a bit of stress with that cord around my neck, obviously pulling tight.

As I went through that rebirthing session feeling the cord slip off over my head; that would have had to happen sometime before or around the time of my birth. I was born at 11:55 a.m. on Saturday morning and the attacks always started subsiding on Saturday afternoons. Perhaps the reason I was transverse lie in the womb in the first place was because of the cord around my neck and I moved to that position so that I could breathe.

As I went through all these experiences I created thoughts that were locked in, that then affected me for my whole life. I have worked through many of them but there will always be things that can still pop up to be addressed and that is because as long as we live here on this planet, my sense is that we will always be a work in progress, continually learning.

Some of those thoughts I created included being abandoned and rejected, controlled and manipulated (forceps and the binding) to name a few. It doesn't mean to say that is how it was; it is simply what I decided and once those thoughts were locked in, along with the corresponding emotion, all it ever needed was the triggers to set things off. i.e., the asthma attacks.

There are a couple of other things which may help to tie some of my findings together. When I was a teenager my mum actually told me that when I was born my dad had wanted a boy. I was stunned and found that hard to believe as my dad and I had a great relationship. She told me that she always thought I knew somehow even though there was no way I could have known, because from the time I came home from the hospital I followed my dad everywhere with my eyes and his name was my first word. As soon as I crawled, I followed him everywhere and more so once I started walking.

We had a small hobby farm so I was up early a lot of mornings when I was little so I could sit and watch him shave and then join him to tend to the animals before he left for work. He was an avid gardener and I spent hours in the garden with him, singing his favorite songs to him.

I was a real tomboy, climbing trees, fences and gates; all the things boys do. On Sundays he would take my brother and I on walks around the countryside and he taught me to love and appreciate nature and the environment. If he suggested trying something I would act on it right away; it was his idea for me to play tennis and I took to it immediately. Looking back now I can see that it does appear that on some level I was aware of what he wanted and I tried to prove to him that having me was just as good as having a boy. What came to me during the Rebirthing sessions showed how I came to those conclusions. My mum also said that although he had wanted a boy, I stole his heart from the very beginning and he was always very proud of his little girl.

Then there was the first asthma attack upon being presented with a brother. My dad also told me at our last get together that it was made clear to me that the new baby might be a boy but I was adamant I wanted a sister; nothing else. I was sent to relatives while my mum was in hospital and for some reason was told there that I had a sister. My parents never knew why this was done and they thought this caused my reaction. That may have been part of it. However, knowing now what was in my subconscious from my own birth about my dad wanting a boy, who knows what my reasoning could have been. Here was that boy they wanted; would they even want me now and this takes one back to the original thought pattern I came across at the beginning of my search, about not wanting to be here, not wanting to be alive. Finally, I could make sense of it all.

At that point, after all the rebirthing, I thought I had all the answers I needed but there was one more major piece to the puzzle and it came along many years later when I had a chance to do a water Rebirthing, in a warm pool, which simulated being in the womb. I was face down in the water using a snorkel to breathe and the facilitator was right beside me to lend a hand if need be. I did wonder if I would be able to do such a session as it did not feel natural.

However, it turned out to be very easy and I didn't have to go too far into the session to have activation. I realized right away that I was back in the womb and then all these thoughts started to pop into my head, which I knew were my mother's, to the effect that she wasn't ready to be a mother and she didn't know whether she really wanted to be a mother. I became very distressed and came up out of the water sobbing about how my mother didn't want me either. The facilitator was able to help me through the process so that I was able to integrate and finish the session in a peaceful, relaxing way.

Perhaps doing a session in water somehow activates differently as I had been doing sessions now for a few years and yet it took the water session to get this realization around my mother. Then again, I may not have been ready to deal with it until then or it could be that being in Australia (which is where I did the water Rebirthing) somehow made a difference. The energy of that country is where my journey started and it may have needed that vibration to surface. I was pleased to have this kind of verification because, up until that point, I had no idea how my mother had felt about having a daughter or even having a baby for that matter. As she became ill and passed away quite quickly when I was in my early twenties, there were a lot of things that we never had the chance to talk about.

Note: Something that needs to be addressed here is the fact that on a couple of occasions Rebirthing has been reported on the news in very unfavorable situations and some may be aware of those stories. My experience with the therapy was completely safe and I would not have been a part of it if I had any misgivings at all about the process.

Chapter 9

CHILDREN AND aSTHMA

asthma in children seems to be on the increase these days. There is also a lot of concern about the environment being a big factor around this increase as well as the food we eat and the additives in it. While it is true that our air quality may not be as pure as it used to be (but much better than back in the coal burning days) and there does seem to be a lot more irritants in the air that are problematic for our breathing, is it just these things that are the cause or perhaps they are just triggers, with the cause being something else; something that may be on the inside.

If you have read through the book to this point, you will be aware of all the different avenues I took, looking for answers. However, if you're just jumping to this chapter to fast track information because you have an asthmatic child or know of one, you may find yourself becoming annoyed with what seems to be a lot of mumbo jumbo or as a friend called it years ago, "woo woo" stuff. I went "outside the box" so to speak, in my quest for ideas and theories and to get results, for both children and adults.

So often parents are not comfortable with doing this; my parents wouldn't have been. But life has changed a lot since then as have medicines and treatments. Today there is so much more information that can be accessed by so many different avenues and we, as a people, are more aware and willing to try different things and the biggest thing is that no parent likes to see their child suffering and not being able to live their life to its fullest capacity.

Children may have asthma for all sorts of reasons. Perhaps they were born with it or it came on gradually while they were still young, as a result of colds and/or lung problems like bronchitis, or like me, it may have just appeared, triggered by some event.

Let's look first, at a baby that has asthma. All the information I found around the reasons for asthma at that point in one's existence showed that on some level, the baby does not want to be here and has a fear of the world and life itself. For some reason they feel unwanted, unwelcome or even rejected. There was also a suggestion that the baby gets these feelings from the mother which makes sense seeing as they spend nine months in the womb. There may be any number of reasons for how or why a mother thinks as she does during pregnancy and it doesn't mean the baby picks up every single thought either. This is just a reference for you to look at, to get you thinking about any and all scenarios.

What if there is a history of asthma in the family?

Well, that would explain the wiring in place but the trigger to get it started may originate elsewhere. There are many areas in which to look. Reflect on the birth of the child and try to remember if there were any problems around breathing or possible suffocation while in the womb; anything around breathing restrictions during the birthing process itself, and finally, right after being born.

Examine what was said before baby arrived; what the

mother was thinking all through labor and at birth and right afterwards. From my experience I know the baby is very aware of everything that is going on and can pick up its mother's thoughts very easily and can also hear whatever is said in the room at the time too. It used to be thought that babies had no cognizant awareness of anything until well after they were born. My mother, when she told me of my forceps episode, said how thankful she was that I was too young to feel it or have any memory of it. Little did she know! The experience was still there; just sitting in my subconscious.

Another thing to consider is the fact that your thoughts may not come across to the baby in the way you might think they do. Perhaps you had a thought that was meant to be a joke but it doesn't mean that baby picks it up that way. We have no control over how someone else decides on a thought; what it means to them and therein lies the crux of the matter. As we are all individuals, so shall we think? This is all just information to help you understand a little more clearly, how there may be things that impact a baby from a very early stage. In all the Rebirthing sessions I have done I have never had a session where I was aware of any other experiences during that nine month period other than at the time of my birth. However, there may be people out there who have done Rebirthing sessions and had all sorts of realizations during that time period. I can only relate how it has been for me in my experience.

An example I can give around possibly picking up thoughts at birth is in the case of my son. He was born quite quickly and laid across my stomach. I was ecstatic and started raising my arms up towards him. At that moment a nurse yelled, "Don't touch him". I was so surprised I actually jerked and put my arms back down. From that day forward I had a terrible time holding my son; he was great with his dad, grandparents and everyone else; falling asleep on their shoulder or in their arms, but if I held him for any length of time at all, he would cry and if I didn't put him down, go to screaming. It was very embarrassing at times and back then I could not think of any reason why it kept happening. As a young child, he also did not like any affectionate touching, like hugging and cuddling, especially with me and rarely sat on my lap and if he did, he jumped off as soon as he could.

This situation continued until he went into school and it gradually changed, on his terms and I allowed him to dictate what he felt comfortable with. I really did not understand why he wouldn't accept affection but I knew enough to be patient and not to try and force the issue. It wasn't until I did my own Rebirthing and discovered how everything that happens at birth can have a profound effect on the baby, that it dawned on me how the yelling incident at his birth may have been the reason for his 'don't touch me' attitude. It didn't help either that within twenty four hours of his birth he had to go into an incubator because of an infection and jaundice and was there for over a week.

Possibly that re-enforced the fact that he wasn't fit to be touched. Today, as a man, he says that although he cannot say he has no problems around giving and receiving affection, he is much better at it since having done Rebirthing sessions while living and working in Australia.

Did 'don't touch him' create a negative thought pattern for my son?

There is no way to prove that it was anything other than what it sounded like; a comment made at the time which was an appropriate one considering the circumstances. At that moment I may have had a thought which he picked up; something like "what's wrong with him" or "there's something wrong with him". I don't remember what went through my mind at that time but both my thought and the statement said out loud could have been picked up by him and locked in and he began a certain path as to how he reacted to touch, from me and maybe from all women, from that day forward. Most babies respond to being held and cuddled and it is part of their bonding with their parents. No-one else, family or friends, had any problems while holding him and as I was thrilled beyond words with my baby boy, it wasn't a case of him responding to an agitated or worried mother or someone who didn't want him. He was planned and we were excited about his arrival.

There is also the opposite experience as in the birth of my grand-daughter who was a difficult birth and Caesarian. Right after she was born the doctor handed her to my son and said 'she's perfect' and today that little girl is an expression of that in her natural self-confidence which is wonderful to see. No doubt many other babies have had the same positive beginnings as well.

There is one other area to look at with babies and also young children and this is where people sometimes find it too much of a stretch to even consider such a thing or it may be against their religious beliefs; any number of reasons can come up in this instance and it is understandable. I had no idea about such a thing until I actually experienced it. I am talking about past lives.

What if the asthma comes from an unresolved past life experience?

There have been reports of young children knowing accurate details about another country, other than the one they have been born into, as well as also knowing people and their names which, upon investigation, it has been discovered actually existed; just in an earlier time period. Once again, we come to that idea of having an open mind about everything. Thinking back to my regression sessions, one of the breathing restriction experiences I had, came from a past life.

How is asthma different in children?

My searching over the years kept turning up information around control with children; that asthmatic children often live in controlling situations where one or other of the parents are very controlling. Both my parents were controlling which I put down partly to the fact that they both served in the military and that lifestyle produces a certain amount of rigidity. Quite a long time ago I actually told a mother of an asthmatic child about this theory of a controlling parent or parents. She thought about it for a minute or so and then agreed, saying that she was aware that she was controlling and could see how it might have affected her child.

Parents are not consciously aware that they are controllers. They see themselves as being caring when in actual fact the child feels like it is being suffocated or smothered. This, in turn, means the child starts to learn how to control; in order to survive. I worked hard at having some control over my environment when I was a child. As an adult I was also a controller, just like my parents. My son felt suffocated all his growing up years and now, since I've done so much personal growth work, I can see how stifling his life was at times because of my constant need to have control over everything and everyone in my environment, at all times.

Some of the other things I found listed as causes for asthma were suppressed grief and underlying sadness which were linked to loss and deprivation. If a child has a favorite family member or friend die while they are quite young, it may be a factor or the sadness could just be connected to a thought pattern they took on at birth, for whatever reason. When a loved one dies, the child is often told that 'so and so' has gone to heaven and they are now happy and that is the end of it. Except that it isn't really. Children do see death differently from adults I think, but there is still the emotional quotient around that loss; children need to be encouraged to talk or cry or do whatever it takes, to learn that expressing emotions is healthy and this is especially true for asthmatics.

What about children that live in challenging environments?

Not everyone lives in a fairytale existence, although at times we may have all wished that we did. Some households can be challenging for children for one reason or another. asthmatics, according to my findings, tend to have overdeveloped consciences and take on guilty feelings for whatever seems wrong in their environment and that guilt leads to a subconscious need to punish themselves and along comes an asthma attack; bit of a vicious circle actually.

There was an alcohol problem with my mother in our household that started around the time I began elementary school and subconsciously it became my problem which I tried to fix and as it went on for years it caused a lot of chronic fear and anxiety in me which is something else that is prevalent in asthmatics. Upon looking back I realize that my coping mechanism for my situation was Sports and it served as a valve to release tension that would build up in my body. However, when that need was no longer there, I stayed trapped in over-drive due to subconscious patterns still running the show. We can also sometimes become over achievers trying to make up for those deficiencies in our environment, even though we didn't create them. This is just something else to consider when trying to create a history or a life picture for anyone you know who is an asthmatic, whether they be child or adult.

Sometimes a geographic move will help asthma disappear,

especially if the family does not go along. This is where the so called 'honeymoon' period comes in. If, or when, the child leaves home, the asthma often stops and may never come back. In others, it can return in a few years or later in life. In my case, once I started working and the bonds of control within the home environment were loosened, I stopped having the week long attacks and when I left home and moved away, the asthma stopped altogether.

If the asthmatic goes into a similar situation to the one they experienced when younger, such as a controlling marriage or work situation, the asthma may once again surface and this can happen without the asthmatic realizing it. Patterns established early on in life are recognized on a subconscious level and we naturally gravitate to them even if they are not good for us, because it is comfortable and because it is what we know.

This is why the asthma resurfaced for me after a few year in Canada. I went back into the same controlling situation that I had been in as a child, only this time it was in a marriage and I didn't recognize it for many years. I must say here that there is no blame to be attached to the situation. No-one can control you unless you allow it, which I did at that time. After all, it's what I knew and the pattern was familiar to me even though it wasn't healthy.

Everything I've written here is information I came across through all my avenues of researching; from reading articles and books on holistic health, attending talks on the same subject and also from my own life experience. Children are very resilient and deal with whatever comes along as best they can and no-one, not even a parent, unless they are asthmatic themselves, can ever imagine what a child goes through during an attack.

There was an occasion that gave my father the experience

of what I lived with as a child. He was never an asthmatic in his lifetime but did have hay fever. During the winter he had bronchitis for several years when he was in his fifties but after my mother passed away he didn't get the bronchitis any more.

About eight months before he passed away he had his first ever asthma attack which landed him in hospital. His doctor was amazed as the onset of asthma is not common at eighty one years of age. Dad phoned me after he went home from the hospital. He wanted to apologize for the way he and mum had treated me when I was younger and struggling with the asthma. He'd had no idea how bad it was for me but now he knew how scary it was and fighting to breathe was the worst thing he had ever experienced in his life and he wondered how I did it for so many years and survived. It was such a shock for him to actually have that experience and he admitted that he'd had no idea of the severity of the situation that I was dealing with during each attack. Of course there was nothing to forgive; they were only doing what they thought was the best thing to do back then. You can only work with the knowledge that you have at any given time.

Chapter 10

ALLERGIES

This is a huge subject because every spring it seems that more people contract allergic reactions to the environment. The pharmaceutical companies are making a fortune on people who are constantly buying products to get relief and to control the symptoms, not to mention the tissue companies who also get their slice of the pie.

There are many things to look at with the ailment and it may help to break it up into two separate areas of hay fever and allergies, as the thought/emotional causes are a bit different for each. If you have found some of my ideas hard to believe so far, get ready to be even more dumbfounded. I'm not going to pretend it is all about medication because I believe it isn't. Once again, we need to go inside the body and find the cause.

All the physical reactions are outward manifestations of inner turmoil on some level and they are how the body tries to get our attention. However, in most cases, instead of looking for the cause, we medicate ourselves instead and yes, that is a short term solution. It isn't permanent though because in dosing ourselves with pills and sprays etc., we have only suppressed the reactions or triggers and they will keep rising to the surface continually and in some cases, may even become more severe.

Let's look at the hay fever first.

This complaint seems to affect every other person, especially at spring time. If I had five cents for every time someone has told me they have hay fever due to the pollen in the air, I would be rich; it seems an almost chronic situation. Pollen, as it turns out, is not new. It's been around ever since trees starting growing on this planet and the process occurs every year, without fail, during the spring months. It seems to be the human reaction to this annual happening that has changed. For some reason, it now plays havoc with our system.

Let's stop looking to blame something outside of ourselves and look inside, to where the causes are residing, just waiting to be triggered. If we look at it holistically, hay fever is all about emotional congestion and being caught up in hurts from our past which have caused chronic grief. There is also a feeling of being unloved and not feeling safe. People will often disagree with this statement immediately and go on about their happy childhood and perfect parents and so on. That is not what this is about; not directly anyway. Everything may have been perfect for you, at a conscious level, but that is not where you are going to find answers. The answers lie in the subconscious and we don't go there when we are consciously thinking. This is not about blaming; it is about discovering what thoughts/emotions you locked in at a certain point in your life, around some incident that may have been minor to anyone present at the time but to you, the child, it was catastrophic. As children we do not reason; we think and feel on a very different level from our parents and adults so we can be really hurt by something that did not even register in the adult's mind. This is what we are talking about; these things that, for whatever reason, have been a source of pain and bringing them out will begin the healing on the outside.

The other buried mental/emotional pattern that is often associated with hay fever is guilt, which is tied into the conviction that one deserves persecution. When I first came across all these explanations, none of them made sense to me. However, the more I learnt as I went along, the easier it was to see how some of these thought patterns related to me.

Chronic grief was one pattern that was a huge one for me, along with feeling unloved. These were locked in as a result of the trauma around my birth and other incidents and then were triggered when my body reached its limit as to how much suppression it could take.

All the different illnesses sometimes have multiple thought patterns as cause factors and I have found that, in some instances, I didn't have all the patterns mentioned, but one or two definitely fit. At other times, I would discover later on that a pattern I hadn't seen as one pertaining to me at the beginning, now did. As I went deeper into my healing, more things became obvious.

The final avenue that may be worth following up has to do with hay fever always re-occurring each spring while the rest of the year one is hay fever free. Perhaps, somewhere in your lifetime, there was an event or experience that left an emotional wound and it happened during the spring months. After the original hurt was locked in, there is a good chance that every spring after that, the wound would be re-opened by the release of pollen into the air; the pollen being the trigger.

Thinking about past lives may also be relevant here too as it could be something brought forward to complete this time round. The past life idea may not be anything you are comfortable with and that is okay; I do mention it throughout the book because that is where I found some of my answers and without opening my mind to that possibility I may not be where I am today.

Sometimes people think back through their lives and say

nothing traumatic ever happened, but you have to remember that you are thinking back on it now from an adult's perspective and more than likely, you were not an adult when it first occurred; you were a child and so it can be the simplest thing. For instance, a big dog running towards a little child can seem terrifying to them whereas the adult standing beside them, three feet taller, with a totally different perspective of the dog and its size, just sees a friendly dog coming to say hello.

My history with the hay fever as a child was that it generally went into an asthma attack every time. When I reached the teenage years I started having a day long hay fever attack which was exhausting. Sneezing at least 200 times in a day uses up a lot of energy. These were not seasonal either as I had them all year round. They were always on a Sunday, but not every Sunday and every Monday after one of those bouts my mouth would break out in fever blisters (*aka* cold sores).

It took a lot of research to discover what this all meant and it is something I still think I am working on as it doesn't feel like I have totally figured it out as occasionally I will get a day of sneezing, without the fever blisters, so that is progress. When this does occur I check in with myself and go over what is happening or has just happened in my daily life to trigger, what is for the most part, an ailment that normally no longer surfaces.

As it is still able to be triggered means there is still some pattern there that needs to be addressed. As I have done well so far with the asthma, it is just a matter of time before I am able to get to the root cause of the hay fever. As I mentioned earlier on in the book, there was a problem in the family with my mother and alcohol so Sundays were often stressful because of that. There was always a feeling of being smothered and controlled as my life was restricted to being at home to prevent or solve any and all problems that arose from this situation and that triggered all the birth and past life traumas.

The fever blisters are all about speech. They are a result of being angry and having a fear around expressing those words of anger. During researching I found it was said to be anger at someone of the opposite sex but perhaps in my case it was both as there was anger at my mother because of the drinking but there may have been anger at my father too, for not taking charge and leaving me, the child, to deal with the problem. Explaining all this may help someone in their search to find answers as often we do not see how certain situations in our childhood had an effect on us.

There are people who are prone to just hay fever attacks and if they are lucky, only during pollen season but there are others who have allergies and even though they may be triggered a lot more during the spring months, they are plagued most of the year round, reacting to any number of triggers. So let us take a look at allergies.

What causes allergies?

There are many things that are triggers for allergies and they include skin irritations, insect bites, food, medications and chemicals, just to name a few. There are also the hay fever triggers with animal dander, dust, feathers and grasses being on the list. Allergic reactions seem to run in families too. Over 50 per cent of allergy sufferers have other family members who are allergic but what triggers them can vary. It was my father and brother in our family and although I don't know what my father's triggers were, I can remember the marathon type sneezing fits where he would have twenty or more sneezes in a row. My brother has had allergies since childhood and dust is one of the main triggers for him. For relief he used to lie down in a cool dark room until it subsided and today he uses antihistamines to help the condition.

When we go inside to look for the cause, there are many facets to look at and because this is on the subconscious level most times, it's not always immediately obvious how any of the thought patterns could be a factor. Letting go of an allergy involves letting go of all grievances and devastations and allowing the body to feel all the emotions, especially anger and aggression which seem to be linked to this ailment.

Who are we allergic to?

It is easy to understand that the body is experiencing internal conflict of some sort and it is a matter of discovering the source. My research uncovered proposed thought patterns that indicated it all started in childhood and that makes sense if you think about it and although it is life we are really allergic to (on some level we do not want to be here), we transfer that reaction to people or a person. From then on, we react to them, instead of interacting with them.

That internal conflict can be that there is a love for a person, while on another level there is resentment felt because of an emotional dependence they feel to them at the same time. This is normally someone in the immediate family. There is a feeling that if you behave according to that person's expectations, then you will be truly loved.

Following on from this is the idea of non-acceptance at an early age, rejection, neglect and/or trauma that affected the initial emotional development. There may be a longing for the mother's love or even that of a stand-in.

Who was I allergic to?

For the first little while I wasn't even looking for a person because I was sure it was all connected to my birth, which was partly right and from there I moved to thinking it was maybe my birth and also my dad. But that wasn't quite right either.

Further searching and a water Rebirthing session that took

me to my birth showed that as well as putting out the thought about my dad being disappointed at my birth, my mother also had doubts about having a child or even wanting one. So, here were two parents who I decided didn't want me. Looking back, my life was one of trying to be what I thought my dad wanted me to be and also what I thought my mother wanted as well, to please her. I mentioned the hay fever starting in my teenage years and that was triggered I think by an incident when I was fourteen. I was going to stay with friend for a holiday and went to kiss my mum goodbye when she raised her arm to prevent it and said, "You're too old for that now". At the time I was very hurt by her actions. I never forgot the incident and as Sunday hay fever started soon after that I think the two were tied together; I had reached my limit for suppressing emotions around rejection.

Some further information I found suggested that the love the child needed or felt it needed was not there for them, for whatever reason and this may have led to a lot of unexpressed grief. As the mother is the first connection a child has in this life, this maybe where all the trouble starts and once locked in, just needs the outside triggers to set it off. This certainly fit in with my scenario and made perfect sense.

This is not to say that mothers are or were lacking in some way or that they are to blame. Without them none of us would be here. Remember that healing the whole body is taking responsibility for ourselves which means there is no blame being aimed at anyone, at any time. The soul always chooses; there are lessons to learn while we are here and whatever happens, is what happens. This is all just about gathering information to look into and check out and any discoveries made along the way that can help clear up a condition is a blessing.

Some of the other thought and emotional patterns

uncovered which may be helpful are that there is a lack of self-worth and a denial of one's own power and a fear of letting anyone inside their personal boundaries. Being easily intimidated can also be a clue along with being defensive and overly sensitive. These may take a bit more work to uncover as so much is not obvious to us and our initial reaction to most of what we come across, at first, can vary from thinking this is a lot of rubbish, to outright denial. I went back and forth a lot in my journey until, through continual researching, I began to open up more and to see myself as I really was.

One other thing that I came across and this could be a big one in a lot of cases is that if the parents had opposing views in a number of areas and this was acted out around the child, this may have been a cause for conflict within the child and as we know, that conflict, when it reaches critical mass inside, has to show up somehow on the outside, in the physical.

Are there specific thought patterns linked to certain allergies?

I did find a few that provide some information which might match up for some people. Food allergies: Maybe it is difficult to experience pleasure around things that are good and enjoyable.

Dust/animal allergies: There could be an intolerance happening with another person or a persistent feeling of easily being attacked. It is not possible to change others but we can always change ourselves and that will reflect in their reaction to us.

Allergies may also be a residual of past life traumas. If a death was as a result of an accident involving, say a horse; then this life may produce an allergy to horses and it is there to be worked through in this life. This is not a given of course but it is a possibility.

My allergies to animal dander disappeared after my regression sessions when I experienced both the strangulation in the past life and the strangulation in the womb in this life.

One book that I researched had a lot of information that was fascinating and it was called Allergies and Aversions by Michael J. Lincoln, Ph.D. It lists allergies to almost anything you can think of along with the psychological meaning of each. They all involve family dysfunction of one kind or another with a lot of it maternal and about rejection.

Reading that brought together the information that I had come across continually in my search about there not being a family on this planet who isn't dysfunctional on some level and because of the varying degrees of it, some families appear to have it all together more than others and that does seem to be reflected in our society today.

There may be much more information out there as today we have many more resources available than there was when I started on my journey. The more information you have the better equipped you are to find answers to your condition.

Chapter 11

FORGIVENESS

Forgiveness is a component of healing that is often overlooked, but it is an important part of the process. If we loved ourselves and others, forgiveness would not even be an issue.

The ideal way would be to operate from being in the moment with the belief that everything is perfect and at the same time be able to see that perfection in everything and everyone.

However, to get to that point, there is a lot of suppressed emotions like anger, guilt and resentment to release as these have been building up in our body since we were born. When the past can be released, then forgiveness can happen.

It is important to remember that illness comes from a state of unforgiveness and one can usually work out who needs to be forgiven, along with the self. In my case it was my parents and after doing the family history it became evident how these two were struggling with their own pain and hurt. In actual fact, they did a great job bringing up children in spite of their drawbacks. Therefore, it was easy to do the forgiveness when I pieced together the whole picture.

There are many misconceptions around forgiveness but once on a healing path and being able to release past hurts and grievances from the body, it is possible to go beyond the ego conditioning to see the innocence, love and perfection of those with whom we had those original interactions.

When forgiveness is done, there is acknowledgement that a wrong occurred. The emotional hurts of the past are put behind us and there is acceptance that both parties are people who made a mistake. This does not mean that you excuse or condone the behavior and depending on the situation, further contact may not happen, but any anger and resentment there was around the wrong has been resolved and you can move on.

True forgiveness comes from the heart and must be felt; it happens on the inside after releasing the painful emotions and letting them go as hanging on to them is a waste of our thinking power. We have to accept completely that the past is gone; nothing can change what happened. Now, do we want to hang onto all that deadwood and let it drag us down or be forgiving and actually release all the stuck energy being held in the body?

Quite often, forgiving is connected to the 'other' person but it's really about us making peace with ourselves and it is very important as our criticisms, judgements and anger towards others came only as a result of our own suffering. This is a big realization that many struggle with because it means accepting that we alone are responsible for all our thoughts, feelings and actions. Forgiveness gives us freedom and healing which is a real gift; a gift of love – to ourselves.

Forgiving others is to accept them and let go. On one occasion I complained to my mother about an incident with one of my playmates and she told me to imagine walking in their shoes for a day and living their life. I realize today that it was very insightful of her to have me do that because it changed my whole perspective of the situation. I was being asked to look at the whole picture rather than just the role I was playing and to let go; to accept my playmate without any judgement.

There are other ways to look at forgiveness and one is to see that all that happens to us in our life is divinely orchestrated and we are balancing karmic debt and therefore fulfilling our soul's purpose here on earth. Along with this mindset is the belief that as there are no mistakes, there is never anything to forgive.

Another way to approach it is from the 'mirror image' point of view. When we see traits in others we don't like or witness behavior that makes us uncomfortable, it is because that person is mirroring the same traits that we exhibit and it shows us areas that we need to work on around forgiveness.

It is not always easy to forgive and perhaps clinging to those old hurts gives us an excuse to remain where we are in our development and not move forward. The time may not be right for us or we might not feel ready. Everyone needs to do what is right for them, when it feels right to do so. There is no time limit per se and whenever it happens, that will be the perfect time.

Chapter 12

THERAPIES

There are many different natural and holistic type therapies that can be tried and none of them are harmful or dangerous. At times there is fear mongering happening out there and that is a good example of always needing to have complete control to the point of suffocating the rights of people to make a choice and that is so not right. It is, and always will be, our right to make our own choices. There is rarely only 'one' way to do anything and an open mind is a beautiful thing.

It's also good to remember that natural healing methods have existed for hundreds and sometimes, thousands of years, in many cultures all over the world. Today there are many people who have healed themselves through these natural methods while others have achieved the same result by combining medical and natural techniques. In the past we didn't hear too much about it unless it happened in your region but these days, with the internet, we can access any number of instances where this has happened and in some cases, can even communicate with these individuals to discuss with them how they orchestrated their own healing.

When you set out on your healing journey it is important to find the right practitioner.

What constitutes the right practitioner?

This will be someone with whom you feel totally comfortable and at ease and whom you trust implicitly. That way you will get optimal results from any healing sessions you do with them. In today's world everything is done by email or text but it is better, if at some point, you can actually talk to the person by phone or by Skype. That way you can get a feel for them. If there is any apprehension on your part, then maybe that particular healer is not for you.

When I was looking for someone to do Rebirthing I found a lovely lady but when we talked, something felt a bit 'off' so I went looking for someone else and the person I found was a fit immediately. As soon as I saw her photo on the flyer, I knew she was the one and that was before I even read her spiel; my sessions with her were amazing. Some of the modalities I mention are ones I've tried. Others are ones that other people I know have found successful and still others are ones that I've heard about and the reports I've read have all been favorable.

REGRESSION HYPNOTISM was where I had my first big breakthrough and would be something worth looking into because it gets behind the walls we've put up. When I did Regression the therapist told me that children are not usually regressed until they are over seven years of age as that is when their sense of reasoning comes in and they need to be able to do that, to get results and to understand the whole concept of what they are experiencing.

REIKI is another good hands on healing technique. The practitioner channels energy from the Universe, down through her hands into the client. As we are surrounded by energy all it needs is for the practitioner to have the intent and the client will get what it is that they need during the session. Over the years I have had many sessions and had a lot of "stuck" energy moved out. Sometimes I would have conscious realizations of what I was releasing; other times I would just feel fantastic and totally rejuvenated after the session. Reiki can be done on anyone; at any age and animals especially, respond to this type of healing

REFLEXOLOGY which involves the feet is amazing. Apart from your feet feeling wonderful, there can be helpful results too as a good reflexologist is able to pinpoint in the body where there are energy blockages. The treatments are not painful and this is a wonderful treat to give yourself. I have had several treatments and each time walked away with information that helped me identify the next layer of emotion coming up so that I could carry on with my healing.

HOMEOPATHY which includes the taking of remedies is something else I have tried with great success and I go for regular checkups, just as one would to a doctor. At the clinic I attend the homeopathic doctor has developed a reflexology Software which determines organic imbalances within the body. It is such a help to be able to see what is out of balance in the body as it can then be related to one's mental/emotional states to see how the imbalance can be corrected. One must have patience though, because unlike prescription drugs, these results take a little longer to show up but they really work.

ACUPUNCTURE is also something I tried years ago. I did it just as a tune up for a certain area of the body and it worked well. I know others who have gone because they were very ill and had great results. Even though I have had many needles in my lifetime because of the asthma, these needles were quite different; nothing like a regular injection.

BACH FLOWER REMEDIES are about replacing negative attitudes with positive attitudes. I used them quite a bit many years ago and found them helpful. There are 38 remedies with explanations for each and you can easily figure out which one you need. They help to balance the mental and emotional state of the body.

ANCESTRAL CLEARING is something relatively new that I heard about and have participated in as the sessions are done mostly online. It is amazing and as you would guess, it is all about healing back through the ancestral line. It does work as there is so much we have in our genes that is from all those that went before us. This is an excellent tool for clearing the asthma and anything else, for that matter.

MASSAGE is always good for the body to relieve tension, to relax the muscles and any number of things. Any type of body work is essential because it helps to move stuck energy and when you are on a healing journey and working towards releasing, a massage can be very beneficial. Earlier civilizations were very aware of the benefits of massage and in some instances, it was part of their weekly health regime.

CRANIAL SACREL THERAPY is another healing tool for the body. My first experience was as a result of an exchange with another practitioner but I had such good results I still go every so often and have a treatment; if there is anything needing to be released and near the surface CST will move it out.

CHIROPRACTIC has been an amazing healer for a great many people; we stuff so much 'back' there and releasing it can create big changes. I also know that many asthmatics have had success with this technique. When I was younger my neighbor, who was a chronic asthmatic, started going to a chiropractor and the attacks stopped; needless to say he was ecstatic. I also went to a chiropractor for Corrective work, both in Australia and Canada. That involves traction which straightens the spine (curved through years of hunching over during asthma attacks in my growing years). The results have been amazing; the back and neck have straightened by a whole inch and in doing that, a lot of emotional baggage, stuffed back there, has been released.

BIO/ENERGY/CRYSTAL BED HEALING. Bio Energy is one of the most powerful healings I have had in recent memory. I cannot give you details because it is all on a subtle level or was for me anyway; not everyone may be like that. I always walk out a different person from when I walked in so know that there is definitely an energy shift of some sort happening.

The Crystal Bed Healing is also very powerful and there were physical releases around those healings plus actual things happening in the body that I could feel; like the body was being tweaked; put back into shape. Until this healing I had not had dreams for years; now I am getting them on a regular basis again so that was a big shift.

KINESIOLOGY is amazing as it is a great way to get answers from the body, about how the body is feeling and what is not working when you have a qualified person to work through issues with you. The body never lies and it always knows what it needs to heal.

MEDICAL INTUITIVES are also starting to get recognition. People who have been to them find them quite amazing and very good at picking up what is happening in the body.

SALT CAVE THERAPY is something I have tried a couple times and it is said to be very helpful for asthmatics. It is only in recent times these places have opened up here but I have heard they are more common in Europe. They definitely do help the breathing as I noticed that right away even though I don't have asthma anymore.

It seems to clear and open up the whole respiratory system.

SHIATSU also works. I went for several treatments at one point because of stress and tightness in my neck. It loosened the knots and helped tremendously; again anything that helps the body release is worth trying.

MEDIUMSHIP is something that a lot of people think is fake as they class them as Psychics and they are not. They are not reading the body and feeding information back to you that you already know. They connect with the 'other side' and that is where their information comes from. On my journey I had some amazing readings which I was guided to go and have and the information I received around my health was some of the most helpful I ever received.

MEDITATION is very popular and I find it quite helpful to do regularly. In this fast paced world we live in, it is heaven to just sit and 'be'. When I first started it many years ago I used to have to play slow relaxing music to get myself to relax. Now I don't need the music and often it is during this time that solutions to problems present themselves as simply thoughts coming into my head. It really is one of the greatest things to come to us from the Eastern world.

AROMATHERAPY is amazing. I have been using essential oils for years with great success. They are very good for physical ailments as well as the emotions and with one's mental state as well. I use a burner and as well as using them for my healing I often use the oils as a mood enhancer or as a refreshing aroma for a room. People are always commenting on how wonderful it smells in my home and it is all natural which is very beneficial. If there was one area I highly recommend it would be to learn about essential oils and how to use them. They are subtle, smell wonderful and have great healing properties. They can also be used in soaps, lotions, shampoos and perfumes and can be mixed to create your own particular scent if you decide to make them for yourself.

TRADITIONAL CHINESE MEDICINE is something that must be mentioned as I know so many who have gone this route and had incredible healing. TCM is the oldest professionally administered health care system in the world, being over 2,500 years in operation. Its foundation is based on balance also, with the Yin and Yang.

DANCING is something you might not expect to see here but I mention it because years ago I took friends to open dancing evenings. Music was played and people just got up and danced alone in bare feet; doing whatever they felt like doing. This turned out to be a real personal growth technique and healing in its own way for those who came along because it helped them step outside their comfort zone which they never would have done by themselves. It is also interesting to note that dancing also releases tension in the body and if it is done to the extent where perspiration comes into play, then toxins are also released so there is a twofold benefit to doing it as well as the fact that it is fun.

As I mentioned earlier on in the book, I have done Yoga on and off for years and really enjoy it and many people I have met have sung its praises for all sorts of results. While playing sports for years I found that in both warming up and cooling down some of the exercises were actually yoga poses. Many years ago I participated in a few sessions of Tai Chi. It was relaxing but not something I wanted to do on a regular basis but I have met others who feel their life is so much better because of doing it regularly.

There are other things too, like Pellowah, Acupressure, Ayurveda, Naturopathy, Herbalism, Dream work and Art Therapy. Someone told me that Trampoline workouts can actually be very healing. Although I have never tried Rolfing or Feldenkrais I have heard that these two modalities work very well too. There are many other healing techniques around and new ones come along every so often as well. Just keep your eyes open and be aware. If you are intent on healing, things will come to you.

You may meet someone who will give you some information that you've been looking for or you'll come across a flyer about a seminar that sounds perfect. Books you need to read will find their way to you. Once you put out your intent it all starts to happen and it is an amazing journey.

Many years ago I was walking through the Mall and suddenly found myself standing in the bookstore with no recollection of how I came to be in there. I slowly started to walk in, realizing I must be there for some reason and as I walked down the first aisle a book literally slipped off a shelf and fell at my feet. I could not believe it. I picked it up; figured it must be for me and so I bought it. It was called "Little Miss Perfect" by Megan Boutillier. When I arrived home I read the first couple chapters and thought that, although it was okay, there was nothing outstanding about it. When I read the next chapter I was stunned. It was like someone had looked inside me and really saw me; the hurt me that I had kept hidden all my life. The tears I shed throughout that book helped me release a lot of childhood pain and gave me a valuable insight to myself. You never know where help is going to come from so it is a matter of always being open and ready. I have had a few unusual things happen since I started my journey and it never ceases to amaze me when they appear and I'm also very thankful for the help.

These are just some of the healing modalities out there and there are probably others I have missed. Throughout my journey I have found that trying different types of healing really helps you to move forward. Be guided by what feels right for you.

Every time I hear of something I take note; sometimes I do nothing and other times I instinctively know it is something I need to try. Being open to anything that happens to come to your awareness is the key; to dismiss anything out of hand is to perhaps miss out on a golden opportunity.

Chapter 13

THERAPIES/ REBIRTHING

This technique was so successful in helping me find the "root cause" of asthma that I am going to provide quite a bit of information about it. The whole idea of breathing to heal oneself is natural, easy to do, and it produces powerful results.

Rebirthing (*aka* Conscious Breathing) is a safe technique that facilitates spiritual enlightenment, personal transformation and healing on the mental, emotional, physical and spiritual levels. It's also a process of letting go of the control, getting the mind out of the way and allowing yourself to get in touch with suppressed emotions.

The technique is a simple breathing process where the inhale breath is connected to the exhale breath in a continuous circular rhythm until the energy cycle is completed; approximately one hour. The inhale is gentle and deep, the exhale relaxed; not forced.

What makes Rebirthing different from other healing methods is that the emphasis is all about using the breath to let go of the original trauma without getting caught up in it as one breathes through the emotion. Depending on the trauma there may be more than one emotion to integrate as pain, fear and also anger are often all part of one experience. How they integrate, whether separately or all together, will be the right way for the person involved.

These emotions become locked in the body at the time of occurrence. Faced with an unwanted experience, we constrict the breathing (held breath or shallow breathing) and withdraw energetically, thus reducing the ability to feel any pain at that moment. The pain then becomes suppressed and this contracted energy pattern stays in the body and affects us, on all levels, often showing up as a physical disease.

The first few sessions may produce a variety of experiences and recollections of one's birth can also surface at some point, along with physical sensations of tingling, cramping and numbness. Continued breathing at this time dissolves and integrates the negativity that is surfacing so that by the end of the session one feels very relaxed and experiences a deep sense of inner peace.

When Leonard Orr first developed this healing modality it was done in a warm hot tub to simulate being in the womb. However, it was discovered that this activated too much emotional material too quickly so dry rebirthing was developed. Both ways work successfully but dry Rebirthing is more commonly used and more convenient.

What is dry Rebirthing?

Dry Rebirthing involves lying fully clothed on a flat surface (massage table for example) on one's back with arms relaxed at the sides and you breathe for an hour. It is very simple and non -threatening at the same time. The arms being at the sides is natural as that is a sign that the body is open to healing. Whenever arms are crossed over the body, as most body language experts will tell you, there is an unwillingness to receive whatever comes to you at that point.

An hour might seem like a long time but when I did my first 10 sessions it was the fastest hour I ever experienced and that might have been due to sensations and things that were registering in the body, prior to integration. Over the years I have had sessions that did seem like an hour with not much seeming to be happening but I still enjoyed the whole session and had the peaceful relaxed feeling of pure bliss at the end which is the ideal end result.

Each person's experience is totally what is right for them. For some there is a lot of tears; others cannot stop laughing; it is all about moving the energy, whatever form that takes. There can be intense emotion and early life memories may surface. While some may think that nothing is happening, there is always integration of some sort occurring and it can be on a very subtle level. What we need to know consciously will come up along with the original emotion connected to it and once integrated, it is gone forever. The thing to remember is that there has been suppression going on since day one so it can take a lifetime to integrate all those thought patterns.

Is the breathing always the same?

I have touched on the breathing a little bit but to explain it more fully might be helpful. The breath is *Slow and Full* to start, which is pulling in more breath than you normally would when you are lying down. It gets a lot of energy moving in the body and starts the movement of suppressed material.

When a suppression pattern is activated, the facilitator will move the breathing to Fast and Shallow, which is breathing in and out very fast, similar to the panting breath used by pregnant women in labor. Patterns coming up can be quite intense and this level of breathing helps to integrate while also lessening the intensity. It also helps if the attention is focused on the pattern of energy surfacing and where exactly it is in the body.

If people tend to fall asleep during a session, *Fast and Full* breathing is used to bring them back to conscious awareness so that integration can happen and it also works for those who just drift off and then stop breathing momentarily.

One thing to be aware of is to always relax on the exhale so it is not controlled. The body knows how to breathe as it's been doing it all our lives. Putting more emphasis on the inhale is normal as we do that with any type of exertion but pushing on the exhale is not a normal breathing habit.

Breathing can be done through the nose or mouth and both work. I have done both and prefer the mouth because I do seem to get more activation; even though I have had activation both ways. It comes down to personal preference. And finally there is the area of the body to pull the breath from and that can be from the top or bottom of the lungs. Most of my sessions were from the top and I had successful activations each time.

As you can see, there is a little more to it than just lying down and breathing and this is why it is always advisable to do the first ten sessions with a qualified Rebirther.

You always do the breathing yourself but they guide you through the different stages; keep you on track and are an emotional support as well as answering any questions you might have after the session. Attempting to do it alone with no knowledge, other than hearsay or what you have read on the Internet is not really a good idea. It can result in an intense emotional experience surfacing and without help to integrate it, the newly activated pattern of energy slips back into suppression and until it does, one can go through a rough time emotionally.

Breathing in and out for an hour sounds easy and it is but it is not always possible to stay on track with the breathing. Once activation starts, the "monkey mind" as it is called or the "ego" kicks in and all sorts of things happen to distract away from breathing. There can suddenly be an itch that irritates, the legs gets antsy or the mouth feels dry. This means that a pattern has been activated and there is a desire to move away from it, so as not to experience it. However, this is the time to focus on the breathing completely as well as what is happening in the body in order to integrate the emotion that is now at the surface.

Is there activation in every session?

As each layer integrates, it usually activates the next layer. My initial ten sessions were done once a week and I would not be very far into the session before activation would start each time. The interesting thing is that no two sessions are alike and this is a good thing as it prevents controlling of the process as well as having expectations of how the session is going to play out.

Affirmations are often used with Rebirthing. After each session the facilitator and client work together to come up with the new positive phrase which replaces the old thought pattern that ran the life for so long. That affirmation is repeated as often as possible during the following week until the next appointment when it may be changed to accommodate a different thought which emerges in that session. It is helpful to write the affirmations as well as say them and first thing in the morning is a perfect time to do this; before the mind gets really active.

Doing them in front of a mirror can also be helpful as you are then aware of any physical reactions that are happening and it is possible to work towards having a relaxed, happy look which indicates total acceptance of what is being affirmed.

There may be resistance during this time of sessions and affirmations because we are now starting to run the show and this is totally new territory to enter into. We are being proactive instead of reactive and it can be a bit scary but the end result of a healthy body is well worth the work.

Through Rebirthing it was discovered that a lot of negative thought patterns had their beginnings at one's birth so it is a good thing that there have been a lot of changes and advancements made around the birth experience for a baby in today's world.

When Leonard Orr was developing his new technique to help adults, there was a Doctor in France, Frederick LeBoyer, who was starting to deliver babies in atmospheres that were trauma free. Between these two, huge steps were being made to change, what was for most babies, a horrible way to come into this world. Even knowing all this, it is still important to monitor what is said in the room at the moment of birth and the child always needs to hear the words that will be music to its ears; that it is the perfect gift!

There are no age restrictions to Rebirthing. In fact, young people can often get results much faster as they are able to move through the process with a lot less resistance than adults.

Some benefits from doing the process include sleeping better and needing less of it as well as increased creativity. People will often make job changes that were long overdue and in some instances personal financial situations improve as well.

Consciously breathing is an amazing healing technique uniting the spiritual body with the physical body, letting in wisdom and love and it is a Spiritual Gift!

Chapter 14

HEALING THE INNER CHILD

It was many years ago when I first heard of the idea around healing the inner child and I didn't quite know what to make of doing something like that. Today I know that it can be a wonderful healing process for people. Rebirthing also heals the inner child and that is where I did the bulk of my work. However, I did get a start many years before that, but just a little differently. That was when I discovered there was a little child inside and that early work helped prepare the way for future inner work.

The little girl, or boy as the case may be, is the one who endured the hurt and pain in the first instance and although the body grew up and became the adult, that little child is still waiting, frozen inside from the time of the original hurt, for someone to come and help them.

In the meantime, the adult is out there, unconsciously reacting to life according to those emotional wounds and attitudes. In most cases, they are not aware that the rage and panic they might currently be feeling is not related to the here and now at all. They are on automatic response mode, led by those early experiences; the subconscious is in charge.

Meeting the inner child is relatively easy in that it can

be done through meditation, a guided one or one developed by yourself to connect, or even through simple visualization. Sitting quietly in a relaxed way, with perhaps some soothing music playing in the background to set the scene for the meeting is ideal and it may help to have a picture of the younger self to view beforehand.

Another way to approach this exercise is to work with a therapist and this may be preferable, depending on the early life experiences and the severity of pain and hurt the child may have suffered. The therapist actually re-parents the adult, going back to incidents where the child was initially hurt and responds to them in the way that was required in the first place.

It can require a lot of patience to do this work as sometimes the child wants nothing to do with the adult; they don't trust them and because of the early damage, they might not even be able to express any feelings at first. It may take several connections before the child will even acknowledge this adult in their presence at all. It is a real eye opener to realize the burden one has been carrying around inside for so long.

The very first time I did a meditation, "a meet and greet" as it was called by the person leading the group, I didn't know what to expect. We had been told that the first time there might be nothing; our child may not even show themselves. This was to be our first attempt at holding out the olive branch; to let them know that finally, we were recognizing their existence, after all this time

It was a pleasant surprise to find my little person, but she was sitting in the shadows and would not come out, nor would she talk and she really didn't want anything to do with me. It was interesting to me, that she had chosen to sit in the shadows as I, the adult, am a light person, loving the sunshine and everything to do with light.

After that initial meditation I continued to do them regularly by myself and it was a long slow drawn out affair. It took her a long time to move out of the shadows and longer still before I was allowed to approach her. When she finally spoke she actually yelled at me for leaving her and then she cried. That was quite a pivotal moment as right then I actually felt all the pain she was feeling and had been carrying for so long; we both cried together.

We had many meetings after that going through the process of validating my little girl, letting her speak as much and as often as she wanted and recognizing the loneliness that was such a big part of her life. To this day, I still sit and tune into "my little girl" and we chat about this and that; we are good friends these days.

Every so often we have an inner child day where I go and do things she likes to do; go for a swing in the park, walk along the logs on the beach, walk through puddles on a rainy day; swing from low branches on a tree in the park; eat an ice cream. We love to sit quietly and color and we've even gone to the movies; to a children's animated one of course. Sometimes we will be walking past a park and she spontaneously breaks out and we run in for a quick swing......it is so much fun.

The adult me is now learning to parent my own inner child who is a part of me and because it didn't happen for so long, I have a lot of lost time to make up for. So many years I spent squashing and ignoring her, losing that childlike wonder and awe that we can always retain around life if we stay in touch.

It was years later that I did Rebirthing and put all the pieces of the puzzle together as I was now aware of the feelings that little girl had experienced and as an adult looking back, it was easy to understand the suffering and pain that child endured.

Chapter 15

AFFIRMATIONS

Affirmations have been around for a long time, going back to ancient eastern religious practices and are still used today in mantras and creeds that are continually repeated. In the modern world, they took on a new importance once it was realized how big a part the subconscious and our thinking plays, in relation to our health. Whenever talking is done, what is said is either positive or negative as it is being affirmed and it is done all the time.

By affirming something it means taking charge of the mind and stating or declaring that what is being spoken is the way it is. That is why it is so important to think before speaking; to be sure that what is said is of a positive nature. Negative talk is quite detrimental to our well-being.

Although we do not do it purposely, we are affirming constantly with the barrage of advertising that comes at us, repeatedly saying the same thing; getting the same message across. Sitting watching TV is a good example. During the course of say, an hour, the same ads will play constantly, and on some level we absorb that information.

The same goes for going to the movies. It is all about imprinting the mind and if it didn't work well, companies would not be spending the money they do, to have their advertisements aired. All these ads are affirming that happiness only comes from outside of ourselves and that is why we need to buy their products or secure their services or whatever it is that is being advertised. One good thing is that by taping shows, and cutting out the commercials, a lot of that mind washing is stopped.

Learning and practicing positive self-talk can be very difficult at first and an easy way to start off is to choose just one thing to change and work on that. Be aware of what it is, try and catch yourself before saying it and change it before actually verbalizing it.

This can take some time to change and there is a tendency to give up which is all about the "instant gratification" society we inhabit these days. However, patience is a good thing to have because if whatever is being changed has been a part of the vocabulary for many years, it is probably firmly entrenched and will need time to be retrained to a more positive aspect.

What is "retraining"?

That means taking steps to go from negative to positive and sometimes it is too big a jump to go straight from one to the other and you need to bridge a bit. For instance: if you are a person who is always late and every time you arrive somewhere you re-enforce that by continually repeating the statement "I'm always late for everything", then it might be too much to go to, "I am on time for everything". An easier way to start may be an affirmation that states, "I intend to be on time for everything or "I am working on being on time." Eventually, with conscious effort to arrive on time, the new affirmation will affect enough change to be able to move to "I am on always on time for everything".

Whenever thoughts are changed, there must be a change

in the behavior or belief system to accommodate the shift. Just rattling off words and doing nothing to set the change in motion is certainly setting up for failure. As with all healing modalities, once the intent is set, we must take that first step which will create movement and change.

Affirmations are always said in the present, as in, I am, or I have, so as to program the mind that it is "now" we are making a change; not tomorrow or next week, but in this very moment. It is good to be very clear with the affirmations too. Being too general does not give the subconscious much to work with and disappointment will surely follow when nothing happens.

What kind of affirmation would be too general?

Well, let's say it is around work and the affirmation states "I am having a new career". With nothing else to go on, the mind would have a hard time finding what exactly was being requested. Affirmations must be clear and to the point. I am sure everyone is familiar with the saying "be careful what you ask for". Well, it is true. What you ask for and what you get may be very different because there was not enough clarity in the affirmation that was used.

I made that mistake myself. Many years ago, when I was playing Netball and very much into affirmations I created one to help me achieve a goal I had in mind. What I actually desired was to play for Canada in the World Championships but that wasn't my affirmation; it was "I am now on the Canadian Netball Team" and as I believed whole heartedly that it would happen I did create that, along with a lot of physical hard work on my part to get there. However, that was as far as I went, becoming ill and having to retire from the team before the World Championships. So you see, my affirmation did work, but my wording was only partly correct for what I was actually trying to create and it wasn't until a long time later that I realized my success may have been much better if my affirmation had been "I am now playing for Canada in the World Netball Championships.

It is good to create your own personal affirmations; ones that completely resonate with you. The results will always be better if what is being said feels totally right. If saying the affirmation doesn't produce a feeling of total belief in the words, it may come across as a mixed message to the body and the outcome may be less than satisfactory.

At times, working on two or three affirmations at once can work well. After continued practice it will become easier to work through multiple changes as the body will become used to the routine. It's all about being in charge; being proactive instead of reactive. Having a picture in the mind to go along with the affirmation is another technique that works well. Visualizing each aspect of what you are affirming brings it totally into the "now" and what you can conceive of, you can create. First you see it and believe it and it manifests. People have different ways of receiving information through the senses and this is something that needs to be addressed as well.

How does one receive information through the senses?

Everyone learns in a way that is particular to them or ways by which they have more success at retaining and learning any information that comes to them.

There are Visuals: they like to write it on paper and read it or have the written word on a poster on the wall or even on a card in their wallet. Sometimes drawing a picture of the affirmation also works well and putting it on the fridge where you constantly see it is also very beneficial.

Some are Auditory: they prefer to listen, so recorded information works well as does actually verbalizing the words. Going to talks and listening to talks online also gets good results.

Still others are Kinesthetic: they feel and can visualize along with meditation.

Walking and/or running while listening to tapes can also work. It may be that, for some, only one way will produce results but for others, a combination of one, two or even all three of them will work equally as well. I have always utilized all three together in every instance and find that works best for me.

The preferred times for saying affirmations appears to be mornings and evenings because that has been determined the best time to get the information past the conscious mind. For mornings they can be taped to the bathroom mirror, listened to while getting breakfast, on the desktop or even listened to in the car on the way to work. At night time, right before bed is an ideal time to say them so that the subconscious can work on them during the night. Listening to taped affirmations as you fall asleep is another powerful way to get through on that level. However, repeating affirmations day and night and then spending the rest of the time thinking and speaking negatively is probably not going to give you the results you are looking for. To get changes, the whole outlook must undergo a shift, from the negative to the positive.

When I started using affirmations I did get results and the biggest one that I remember is going on a trip to Mexico. At the time I was asked to go there was no way I could afford it but I decided to plan accordingly, as if I was going. I booked the time off work and then did affirmations as well as visualizations, found pictures of the area and put them up to look at and read up on the area. About two months before we were to book the trip, I unexpectedly came into some money and it was enough for the plane fare and spending money. That was amazing, but when it came to the asthma, I could get nothing to change. My conclusion around that has been that general affirmations can work very well but if there is a long time pattern running that is the opposite to what you are trying to create, the subconscious has the ability to override the positive affirmation, even though we have no conscious awareness of that happening. For me, I needed to go in, discover those patterns, integrate them and then run affirmations after that to solidify the new programming.

Do Affirmations Always Work?

Affirmations are powerful; they do work for me and I love working with them to see what I can create but I know people who say it is rubbish and that they tried it and nothing happened even though they did it for months. Perhaps, like me, there was an underlying pattern that, unless addressed first, would mean there could be no permanent changes. Also, I always truly believed I was going to get the results I was aiming for and quite possibly that has a lot to do with how successful one will be. It was always just a matter of waiting to see how long it would take for my affirmation to turn up in my physical world.

Rebirthing and affirming go hand in hand. When a pattern is located and the suppression integrated, the practitioner usually works with the client to find the right affirmation to use so as to prevent that suppression from re-occurring. Once those old negative patterns are integrated, they can be replaced by thoughts of Power, Wisdom, Love and Truth. That is what we all came in with, but sometimes, from the moment of birth onwards, the negative conditioning took over and gradually we lost sight of everything that represented us.

Shorter affirmations do work best. If the affirmation is too long and not clear, the subconscious cannot get a clear picture of what it is that you are trying to create and so the results will most likely not be what you were hoping for. Short and to the point works well. There are many places to look for affirmations if you are not sure how to say something or what words to use. The internet is a great resource for this type of thing. If you are direct about what it is you are trying to create, the more satisfied you will be with the results.

When I started using affirmations and was told that taping them using your own voice was the most powerful way to get results, I put them on a tape recorder and listened to them non-stop during my half hour drive to and from work and I did this for several years, changing them every so often as was needed and it was most successful. It was during this time that I created my trip to Mexico.

Perform your affirmations with faith, trust and belief and you will get successful results.

Chapter 16

THE FOUR BODIES BALANCED

After all the discoveries have been made and the work done around healing the four bodies, it is important to recap and see how things have changed as regards each body and how it now functions. I'm documenting the changes as an example of how things can look after some of the main work is done. If you decide to undertake a healing journey it may look very different; remember that no two of us are alike.

The Physical Body: It is a lot more relaxed and less rigid with a softness to it that was never there before. When I hug people they feel the warmth of the hug whereas years ago (before the journey started) a friend told me that hugging me was like "hugging a board with boobs" which is not very flattering but she was right; I was very rigid with no "give" in me at all.

A gym workout is still part of my daily routine but now I can easily take a day or a week off without all the negative thought patterns that used to surround that decision popping up and I never go and work out doubly hard afterwards, as I used to do, almost punishing the body for taking time off. Working out before was almost like an addiction.

Now I enjoy it for what it is and listen to the body and

respect its need to work a bit harder of a morning because it feels quite energized or take it a bit easier because it feels tired. I could never do that before.

For as long as I can remember I have never felt really comfortable living here on earth and I never really understood what that meant. It was just that something did not fit or I didn't fit. Doing the Rebirthing unraveled all that for me and it was to do with not knowing where I belonged as those early patterns showed me that I decided neither parent wanted me, so why was I even here. Now I am totally at ease, on all levels, with being here.

The Mental Body: This has greatly improved in that I am a lot more lenient with myself as regards derogatory self-talk, using terms like "cancel cancel", if I catch myself thinking a thought that can be harmful to the body and right away replacing it with a positive one. I am working on allowing others to be as they are, respecting their right to an opinion that differs from mine without trying to convince them otherwise. And the amazing thing is that the body feels better when I am able to do that; proof positive that I am on the right track.

The control issue was a big hurdle for me to overcome because it came from not feeling safe in my environment. Again the Rebirthing and the integration of some childhood patterns have helped me to "lighten up", as they say, as regards to myself.

People were forever telling me to do that and I never understood what they were talking about; today I do. There are still occasions when that "control" issue will be activated as another old energy pattern emerges but now I can often see them immediately and take action right there in the moment.

The Emotional Body: there has been a real shift in this area, from being really suppressed to being open and receptive.

I've learnt to cry and during the course of my journey have filled many buckets with tears as I integrated a lot of grief. I can now feel the excitement that goes with happy events, like preparing to go on vacation or finally securing tickets to attend a favorite concert or show. It feels wonderful and I am more aware of the sensations in the body and enjoy those feelings.

Expressing joy and enthusiasm and being more confident is a lot more natural for me as well and it leads to a more positive outlook on life. The anger can still come out, very occasionally, but it is almost unrecognizable compared to those earlier days.

Sometimes I know right away what is triggering my response but there are times I don't and so have to do some work around finding a particular thought pattern that is still lurking in my subconscious.

Spiritually I have gained a stronger connection with Source which seems to come naturally as the work is done and the negative patterns are integrated; patterns that weakened the connection when they were originally created. Meditation is now a regular part of my life, which means taking time out to listen to Source and that comes after prayer, which is talking to Source.

A habit I have formed is to look for the positive in anything that happens in daily life. I've found it to be a perfect way to move away from the not so positive aspect which jumps out first when something occurs and tries to demand all of our attention. It may take a while to discover the little silver lining that is positive but there is one for every single thing that happens; we just have to find it.

Something else that is helpful and which I've incorporated into the daily routine is writing in a gratitude journal; just one thing each day. It is a great way to get in touch with everything that is a part of everyday life; even the little things that we often take for granted or don't even normally notice. It brings your attention to the *now*, the ideal place to operate from, all of the time. Chanting has also become a favorite thing to do every so often as well as drumming; both of which create a feeling of inner peace and balance.

One thing I've always done that has always felt very spiritual to me is to "be" out in nature, as in walking along the beach, hiking through the forest or meandering through a park and it is even more so if you leave the cell phone at home.

My journey has seen a lot of advancement in myself as a person but there are times when I still get triggered because of being a work in progress and that will be ongoing with constant opportunities to improve and upgrade in my development. It is not simply about finding a problem, fixing it and then that's it. It is a lifelong endeavor and is perhaps why so many shy away from even starting in the first place and prefer the "sleep" state.

One of the most fascinating things about this transformation of self is what happens when one of those former "trigger incidences" occur. The fact is that nothing happens; that is the beauty of it. You wait for that old reaction to surface and when it doesn't, there is such a feeling of euphoria and almost relief too; hard to put into words but so wonderful. Even after all I have been through; with some good times and some very rough patches, I have no wish to go back; back to being asleep. It has been, and still is, a wonderful exciting time of learning and I'm interested to see where this journey will take me next.

Chapter 17

MIRACLES/COINCIDENCES

Miracles can be, seemingly, ordinary events that become extra ordinary by way of how they happen, when they happen and the effect it can have on the people involved. They are usually accompanied by the belief that divine intervention is the cause of such events.

Then there is the other side of the coin that believes that anything out of the ordinary is a coincidence; occurrences that happen together apparently without reason and still there is another idea that there are no co-incidences, just incidences.

In my own experience I truly believe that because my belief about curing the asthma was always so steadfast and so strong I actually created in my life the results that I desired. It would have been nice to do it without the illness part of it but all the learning I had around that in itself was life changing so it was meant to be.

Did I get help in my quest? Yes, I did. I believe there was a much stronger force beyond me, that helped me on my journey and it was there because I had the intent and I took steps to find what I was looking for and I believe we all get that help when we have intent.

Taking that first step is probably the single most important thing we can do towards healing. There is a saying 'God helps those who help themselves'. If you are not comfortable with the religious ideal that conjures up, just insert whatever name has meaning for you. My preference is "Source" since my trip to the other side. However, it does seem that when people start a process of some kind with a clear intent, doors open, ideas come to them, things happen and they get results.

Throughout my life I have had things occur or not occur, as the case may be, that were very helpful and made me very grateful. The sports day when I was a child in elementary school and competed while experiencing an asthma attack was one occasion I am sure there was someone watching over me. In years gone by I have heard and read of many occasions where an asthmatic child has had a severe attack while participating in physical activity and died as a result of it.

On the Friday nights during my week long attack when just taking another breath was agonizing, I had help. On the mantle in our living room there was a statue of the Virgin Mary. I would focus on it, often asking for help. There were a few times when it appeared to give off a light and I would blink, trying to figure out if it was my eyes or did it actually glow. Whatever happened, it was enough to take my mind off my breathing difficulties and get me through the night. As a point of interest: when the family home was burnt to the ground in the Ash Wednesday fires in South Australia many years later, only one or two small items survived the inferno and that statue was one of them; it came out virtually unscathed and my brother still has it in his home.

Many years ago, after the shocking announcement by the specialist that the asthma was so bad that my life was over, I was still reeling a few days later when I kept getting a thought popping into my head about calling this woman I knew that was a very good Medium. I knew that you had to book months ahead to get an appointment and what good was that to me; I needed help right there and then. However, the thought kept coming in so I decided to call. I found out that she had just had a cancellation, right before I called, for the very next day. That reading turned things around amazingly with all the advice I was given about what to do, to facilitate the healing. I saw a helping hand there too, knowing how difficult and rare it was to get in to see that woman on the spur of the moment.

When I was in the coma my family got the call to go to the hospital on the Friday night as I was not going to make it. My son was getting ready to leave with his dad when he had the feeling that he needed to take my little portable tape player and the tape with the subliminal health affirmations on it. When they got to the ICU they were told that my blood pressure was dangerously high and they had done everything they could at that point. My son asked the nurses to put the tape on with the earphones in my ears as I always listened to it and it might help. They did and within a very short time my blood pressure started coming down. My son later informed me that somehow he knew he had to get them to let me listen to that tape. Someone was whispering in his ear I am sure.

Then there was the last final shot that the doctors had, to try and save me. They had been trying every asthma drug they had to stop the attack but nothing was working.

My husband told me later that the doctor came and told him there was just one other drug they could try. However, there was only a 50/50 chance I would make it because the drug could cause heart attacks but without it, they believed I would die anyway. They tried it and it worked; the attack stopped and I came out of it. That drug was the first puffer I ever used; the one I found pulled off the market when I came to Canada because of the heart attack risk factor. I always thought of that puffer as my miracle because it changed my life back when I was a teenager; guess it still was, even then. There is no way to prove that these happenings were anything other than normal events occurring but somehow I don't think so.

When it came time to move from ICU up to a ward, I was told I would be in a six bed ward and I was dreading it as I was barely coping day to day and could not imagine being with that many people constantly. I even talked to my husband about paying to see if I could get a private room but that was not possible. Shortly after that, the call came down; the bed was ready and off I went. To my shock, surprise and relief I was taken to a room with only two beds and I even had the bed nearest the window.

Later that day a cheery nurse popped in to see me and asked why I didn't have a foot board. When you have paralysis of the legs and feet, the feet need to be kept up straight so that dropsy does not occur. She organized all that and off she went and I never saw her again for two weeks. At that time she breezed in again and knew what to do about a skin problem I was having that no-one seemed to be able to get under control.

She knew how to fix it right away and went out to write it on my chart and then she was gone; as a result the treatment she came up with cleared the problem completely and I never saw her again while I was there. She was like a guardian angel, sent to handle two separate incidents that could easily have turned into major issues for me later on.

There was a problem with my mouth being torn due to tubes being too tight when I was in the coma and my face was quite swollen. It was not healing and was getting to be painful. One morning, as I was waking up, I heard a voice in my head tell me I needed to go outside in the sunshine. I had to get permission from the nurses to go outside and they were reluctant to give it at first because they feared another attack. However, they finally agreed and my husband wheeled me out and I sat with my face to the sun. We did that on two weekends, both days, and my mouth healed in that time. Would I have thought to do that on my own even though I love the sun; I very much doubt it. The directives came from some other source.

Once I was out of hospital I was anxious to fly to Australia to see my dad because of what I had seen while out of my body; that he was leaving soon. I was well enough to walk at a slow pace but tired easily. However, I was determined to go so I started phoning around to travel agents to price flights. I could only afford $1,000 and everything was way over that price but as I knew I was meant to go, I had to keep trying.

A day later a company I called told me it was my lucky day as they had just put a sale on a return flight if you could leave almost immediately, between these certain dates and it was only a three week trip. As I only had a small window to get down to see dad because I had to be back in Canada to attend a family reunion in Saskatchewan, it was perfect. The fare was $800 and so I had $200 left for spending money. There was another case of helping hands taking care of what seemed like an impossibility.

All the miracles or coincidences that have occurred have all made my journey a little easier and at times, put a smile on my face. We all need help at some time or another and any time you have a destination in mind that you are determined to reach, it is the perfect time to put out that intent and then follow the leads and all the coincidences that come with that. It makes for an exciting journey and at the end of it, better understanding and better health can be the reward.

Chapter 18

SUMMARY

When I was five or six, I was sitting in the Doctor's office and heard the doctor say,

"Mrs. Jones, there is no cure for asthma". My body went very still, a surge of something shot through me from top to bottom and in my head I started yelling at my mother

"That's not true mummy, tell him it's not true". I don't think, at that point, that I even understood what I was saying but I know I felt a total rejection to what the doctor was saying and I felt very sad when my mother just sat there and said nothing.

That memory never went away and it would pop into my head every now and again and strangely enough I never told anyone about the experience I had. It was many years later before I even began to understand what happened that day. It was like I had a "knowing" on some level, that my condition could be changed. When the "puffer" came out in my teenage years I thought that might be what I was looking for but as it turned out, it was much more complex than that.

From those early beginnings the seeds were sown for being healthy and that is where the belief needs to be. A healthy body is normal; sickness is not a natural state of being. As we are created in God's likeness, I doubt He would see himself as being less than perfectly healthy.

aSTHMA CURED

Throughout my research the same thread ran through and around everything to do with healing and how illness is about a deep separation from Source or God or the Creator; however you see that higher power. After being out of the body I have no doubt about that. Having believed in that higher power all my life, my time 'out there' just re-enforced it even more. Each of us is a wonderful individual and very special, a Divine spark!

Healing is becoming 'whole' again, becoming one with All That Is. It's about balancing the Mental/Emotional, Physical and Spiritual bodies. Having intent is the key to unlocking the door to healing. Be willing to put that thought out there. Know how powerful your thoughts are; look at where you are today and realize that your thoughts have brought you to this point.

Then comes that all important part of doing something physical to get the whole process rolling and that is taking the first step; little baby steps are good and before you know it, the journey is under way. Another thing to remember is that by making that decision to start a healing journey, it doesn't mean you will be so overwhelmed you won't be able to handle it all. I found that in any situation we never get more than we can handle, although at times it feels like a bit of a struggle, but that is usually just our own resistance to something new.

And finally, there is the decision to take responsibility for our lives and everything in it. From "out there" it was a much clearer concept than it is seeing it from inside ourselves. As a society there has been a bit of a slide backwards around "taking responsibility" but with continual growth and change, hopefully the pendulum will swing back to help that development occur.

Something else to remember too, is that age is not necessarily a deterrent either; not unless you decide it is. I was forty two when I almost died and my biggest discoveries came after that time.

This book comes to help you realize you have the power

126

to do much more than you may have ever thought possible and to salute you for getting to this point, to read about the possibility of making changes. Even though this is geared towards asthmatics, these changes can be used for any illness.

Along with stepping into your own power and working on self -healing comes the ability to start loving the self. This aspect is so important and sometimes it can be a struggle just to like what we see, let alone to love it. Initially it was a surprise to discover that I didn't love myself and I had no idea how to go about changing that. It turned out to be something that started to happen automatically as I was able to change those long standing mental/emotional patterns that had formed who and what I was before I started the journey.

My journey is one that has taken a long time and it will be ongoing until I leave this earthly plane. There have been some hiccups along the way but it has never stopped being exciting as I came across a new idea, a new thought, an interesting book or listened to a talk that was inspiring. Learning all about oneself and what makes us function can be a wonderful thing; we are all very special souls having a human experience. Enjoy your journey; wherever it may take you.

THE END

Bibliography

Orr, Leonard D./Ray, Sondra	*Rebirthing In The New Age*
Laut, Phil/Leonard, Jim	*Rebirthing-The Science of enjoying All of Your Life*
Sisson, Colin P.	*Rebirthing Made Easy*
Mandel, Bob/Ray, Sondra	*Birth and Relationships*
Ray, Sondra	*Celebration of Breath*
LeBoyer, Dr. Frederick	*Birth Without Violence*
Ramacharaka, Yogi	*Science of Breath*
Murphy, Joseph	*The Power of The Subconscious Mind*
Hay, Louise L.	*You Can Heal Your Life, The Power is Within You*
Gawain, Shakti	*Creative Visualizations*
Boutillier, Megan	*Little Miss Perfect*
Dyer, Dr. Wayne	*Real Magic*
Jampolsky, Gerald G	*Love is Letting Go of Fear*
Buscaglia, Leo	*Born For Love*

Chopra, Deepak	*Ageless Body, Timeless Mind*
Tolle, Eckhart	*The Power of Now*
Redfield, James	*The Celestine Prophecy*
Leman, Dr. Kevin	*The Birth Order Book*

Author Biography

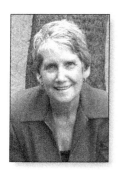

Mavreen was born in Australia and has lived for many years in Vancouver. Holistic or whole body healing has been an interest of hers since discovering Hatha Yoga as a teenager. As a child she suffered from week long attacks of asthma and a lifetime quest to discover the actual cause led her to try many different techniques. After a life threatening attack of asthma, which included an 'out of body' experience, temporary paralysis and six weeks in hospital, she finally came upon a technique which enabled her to connect with the causes and take steps to eradicate it altogether. Consequently there has been no re-occurrence of the asthma attacks since 1990.

Mavreen has also given talks on the importance of healing the whole body to the asthma support group of New Westminster as well the Metaphysical Society in Surrey BC.

aSTHMA BE GONE!

Are you searching for ways to improve or even live *without* asthma?

This book may be your first step towards changing or improving your condition.

Are you a thinker?

Are you willing to change your thinking?

Can you envision breathing freely *all* the time?

If so, the information you read will be exactly what you are looking for as it details how Mavreen changed her condition to be asthma free for the last 26 years. She is very passionate about letting other asthmatics know of her success and how she did it in the hope that others will be inspired to try and help themselves. She has given talks to asthma groups, the psychic society as well as participating in wellness shows as well as a night school course on healing the whole body.

Mavreen can be reached at:

www.asthmacured.ca
mavreenjones@gmail.com
www.influencepublishing.com

CPSIA information can be obtained
at www.ICGtesting.com
Printed in the USA
LVOW04s0811110816

499889LV00018B/98/P

9 780995 251908